CAMBRIDGE TEXTS IN
THE PHYSIOLOGICAL SCIENCES

Editors: R. S. COMLINE, A. W. CUTHBERT
K. C. DIXON, J. HERBERT
S. D. IVERSEN, R. D. KEYNES
H. L. KORNBERG

1 Mechanisms of drug action on the nervous system

Mechanisms of drug action on the nervous system

RONALD W. RYALL

LECTURER IN PHARMACOLOGY
UNIVERSITY OF CAMBRIDGE
AND FELLOW OF CHURCHILL COLLEGE, CAMBRIDGE

CAMBRIDGE UNIVERSITY PRESS

CAMBRIDGE

LONDON · NEW YORK · MELBOURNE

Published by the Syndics of the Cambridge University Press
The Pitt Building, Trumpington Street, Cambridge CB2 1RP
Bentley House, 200 Euston Road, London NW1 2DB
32 East 57th Street, New York, NY 10022, USA
296 Beaconsfield Parade, Middle Park, Melbourne 3206, Australia

First published 1979

Printed in Great Britain at the
University Press, Cambridge

Library of Congress Cataloguing in Publication Data
Ryall, R. W.
Mechanisms of drug action on the nervous system.
(Cambridge texts in the physiological sciences; 1)
1. Neuropharmacology. I. Title. II. Series.
[DNLM: 1. Nervous system–Drug effects. WL104 R988m]
RM315.R9   615'.78   78–5965
ISBN 0 521 22125 0 hard covers
ISBN 0 521 29364 2 paperback

To Audrey

Contents

Preface

In recent years there have been many important advances in knowledge concerning the mechanisms of chemical synaptic transmission, the identification of the neurotransmitters and the mechanisms by which drugs act on the nervous system. These advances have necessitated a change in approach to the teaching of the pharmacology of the nervous system to undergraduate science and preclinical medical students from a basically therapeutic orientation to one which is more mechanistically minded. In giving such courses to students in Cambridge, the author has become painfully aware of the need for an undergraduate text which could fulfil the needs of students in this respect. There are of course many excellent textbooks of therapeutics available but few of them attempt to cope in detail with mechanisms of drug action, especially on the central nervous system, except from rather specialised viewpoints. It was therefore considered to be unnecessary to discuss therapeutic applications in detail in this book, although an attempt has been made to give a fairly balanced account of the physiological basis, applications and mechanisms of action of each class of drugs, within the limitations imposed by the objective of producing a concise account of drug actions in a volume which not only fulfils a need but would also not 'break the bank' of undergraduates.

Advances are occurring at such a rate that some of the concepts which are current today may be superseded tomorrow: this is probably true for any subject that is 'alive' and progressing. However, this does create problems in deciding what to omit and what to include. As far as possible, the basic approach adopted in this volume is to present a coherent 'story' which will enable the student to develop concepts and, perhaps, ideas of his own. Only in this way is it likely that a continuation of progress can be assured and that future medical graduates will not see drugs simply as liquids in bottles to be administered in an empirical manner without understanding to patients with diseases of the nervous system: a reasonable concept, compatible with contemporary information, even if subsequently found to be incorrect in detail, is surely better than no concept at all. Nevertheless, where concepts are relatively insecure, or mechanisms completely unknown, no attempt has been made to disguise this fact in order to present a 'story': such an approach could lead to unjustified complacency.

Abbreviations

ACh	Acetylcholine
ANS	Autonomic nervous system
C10	Decamethonium
C10-TMA	Decamethylene-bis-trimethylammonium
CNS	Central nervous system
CSF	Cerebrospinal fluid
DA	Dopamine
DOPA	Dihydroxyphenylalanine
d-TC	d-tubocurarine
ECT	Electroconvulsive therapy
EEG	Electroencephalogram
e.p.p.	End plate potential
GABA	Gamma-amino-butyric acid
GAD	Glutamic acid decarboxylase
HC-3	Hemicholinium
5-HT	5-hydroxytryptamine
LSD	Lysergic acid diethylamide
MAO	Monoamine oxidase (a mitochondrial enzyme)
m.e.p.p.	miniature end plate potential
NA	Noradrenaline
PG	Prostaglandin
PTP	Post-tetanic potentiation
TEA	Tetraethylammonium

CHAPTER ONE

Introduction

There are two important systems involved in the control of body function, the endocrine and nervous systems. They do not operate independently, although the control of hormonal secretions by the nervous system has been better elucidated than the converse control of the nervous system by hormones. The mechanisms by which drugs modify the operation of one of these control systems, the nervous system, either to produce therapeutically useful effects or to cause undesirable toxic reactions or side-effects, will be examined in the ensuing chapters.

An important feature of the normal operation of the nervous system is that control signals are not only conducted along nerve fibres as action potentials but are transmitted across the junctions between nerve cells as postsynaptic ionic conductance changes, usually accompanied by postsynaptic potentials which serve to excite or inhibit the following neurone in a chain of neurones involved in a particular response pattern or to produce or inhibit activity such as secretion or contraction in an innervated effector organ. These junctions, or synapses, have multiple functions in transmitting information or modifying its transfer between neurones, and collectively form the basis for integration in the nervous system.

The majority of synapses operate by means of chemical transmitters which act as transducers to convert the fairly constant electrical energy of the action potential into a variety of electrical effects upon the postsynaptic cell. Electrical transmission, without the intervention of a chemical transmitter, also occurs to a very limited extent in the mammalian nervous system, but electrically transmitting synapses seem to require a greater degree of gross morphological specialisation than do the chemical synapses.

Fortunately for pharmacology and therapeutics, the diversity of chemical transmitters, of the receptors with which they interact and in the membrane processes which they initiate has made it possible to find and to exploit drugs which often act in a relatively selective way with one or other of these mechanisms. Such selective effects may influence the postsynaptic action of a particular transmitter by interaction with its specific postsynaptic receptor or by influencing one of the many processes involved in transmitter release such as uptake, storage, the release process itself, or the synthesis of the transmitter from precursors.

It seems rather obvious that the most successful drugs are likely to be those which act in a selective fashion either upon a process which is functioning incorrectly or act so as to compensate for dysfunction in another system. Only by selective action is a drug likely to be free from the undesirable effects which usually accompany a therapeutically beneficial action. However, since a particular process is usually common to many nervous pathways, not all of which are equally affected by disease, it is perhaps less obvious that it will be an exceedingly difficult and sometimes impossible task to find drugs with high therapeutic efficacy which are completely free from unwanted side-effects.

Ideally, the development and design of a new drug for a specific application would be aided by a thorough knowledge of the basic physiology of the central and peripheral nervous systems and of the precise cause and effect of the pathological process which has caused the dysfunction. Only rarely is this ideal situation approached and it is significant that many of the drugs in common use, or their prototypes, are of plant origin and their major effects were often known and exploited long before the advent of contemporary physiology, pharmacology or pathology. Serendipity has contributed a great deal to the contents of the modern pharmacopoeia and many of the drugs now used for one purpose were originally introduced for quite another. Nevertheless, the systematic pharmacological study of therapeutically useful drugs has greatly increased our understanding of how such drugs work and has often in the process greatly advanced our knowledge of the underlying basic physiology. The systematic search for new drugs with high efficacy and reduced side-effects has considerably improved the pharmacological spectrum of activity of prototype drugs, even if it has not often directly led to the evolution of new drugs with a radically different mode of action: such a rational development of new drugs with different modes of action must surely await a more complete understanding of the physiology of the nervous system and of the pathological changes which occur.

In the meantime, the treatment of nervous disorders is largely empirical. The alleviation of unpleasant symptoms, perhaps slowing the pathological progression of the disease and prolonging life is a worthwhile therapeutic objective. To cure the disease and reverse the pathological changes which have already occurred is rarely possible and remains a tantalising goal on far distant horizons. Many of the drugs in current use cannot correct the specific abnormality but may produce other changes which can compensate for it. Theories concerning the underlying nature of the disease and which are based upon the known pharmacological actions of drugs which are clinically useful represent useful working hypotheses but are intrinsically insecure. Nowhere is this more clearly the case than in serious mental disease such as schizophrenia, where the mode of action of the neuroleptic drugs seems reasonably clear, but where the lack of clues based on direct evidence leaves the basic nature of the disease beyond our present grasp. In contrast, in Parkinson's disease there are fairly complete data regarding the mode of action of useful drugs, of the chemical and anatomical pathology of the disease, of the normal neuropharmacological anatomy and electrophysiology of the basal ganglia but the precise function of the basal ganglia in motor control remains difficult to assess.

The following chapters will examine how drugs may alter the function of the nervous system to compensate for disease-induced malfunction, for example in myasthenia gravis or endogenous depression, or to produce clinically desirable effects unrelated to any particular dysfunction as in anaesthesia, to cause toxic reactions, as in tetanus, or to counteract such toxic effects, or to have actions which lead to abuse, as with the opiate drugs and psychedelic drugs such as lysergic acid diethylamide (LSD). So far as is possible, the basic philosophy will be to match a drug mechanism to a physiological basis and, where appropriate, to a pathological change.

CHAPTER TWO

Pharmacology of the neuromuscular junction

PHYSIOLOGICAL BASIS

It can be expected that the most precise determinations of the mechanisms of drug actions can be made upon physiological systems which are anatomically and functionally simple and which can be functionally or physically isolated from the whole organism. In these respects, the junctions between motor nerves and skeletal muscles would appear to be almost ideal and the neuromuscular junction is a good place at which to begin a study of the ways in which drugs can influence the process of synaptic transmission.

Anatomy

The majority of mammalian skeletal (striated) muscle fibres are focally innervated by axon terminals, forming on each muscle fibre a single synaptic junction at the motor end plate. A motoneurone in the ventral horn of the spinal cord gives rise to an axon which may branch within the muscle to form motor end plates on each of a number of muscle fibres, together forming a motor unit which behaves functionally as a single entity (Fig. 2.1). The large, extrafusal muscle fibres which generate the major component of the force developed in muscle contraction are innervated by large α-motoneurones through myelinated A fibres. The muscle fibres of the muscle spindles are innervated by the small γ-motoneurones giving rise to small myelinated γ-fibres of motor nerves.

Some muscle fibres in amphibia and in birds, e.g. the rectus abdominis in the frog and the biventer cervicis muscle in the chick respectively, have multiple nerve endings upon them and this results in important differences in their physiological responses to nerve stimulation and in their pharmacological responses to drugs.

4

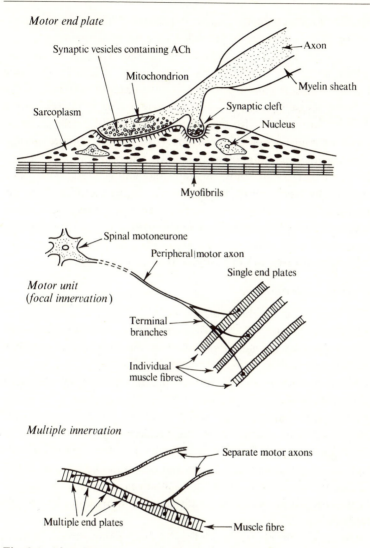

Motor end plate

Synaptic vesicles containing ACh

Mitochondrion

Axon

Myelin sheath

Sarcoplasm

Synaptic cleft

Nucleus

Myofibrils

Spinal motoneurone

Peripheral|motor axon

Single end plates

*Motor unit
(focal innervation)*

Terminal branches

Individual muscle fibres

Multiple innervation

Separate motor axons

Multiple end plates

Muscle fibre

Fig. 2.1. After Couteaux, R. (1958) *Exp. Cell. Res. Suppl.*, **5**, 294.

Techniques

Neuromuscular transmission can be investigated *in vivo* by stimulating the motor nerve at some convenient place after cutting it centrally and recording the resulting contractions by means of a force-displacement transducer. Alternatively, muscle action potentials can be recorded as electromyograms by electrodes inserted into the body of the muscle. Drugs may then be administered systemically by intravenous injection or more localised effects can be ensured by intra-arterial injection.

Some muscles can also be easily removed from the whole animal, complete with an attached nerve, e.g. the sciatic–gastrocnemius preparation of the frog or the phrenic nerve–diaphragm preparation from mammals. The preparations can then be used *in vitro* to study the physiological processes of transmission by electrical or mechanical recording methods, with the added advantage that drugs may now be administered to bathing fluids in accurately known concentrations or may be applied iontophoretically to localised areas of muscle fibre membrane whilst monitoring the mechanical or electrical responses.

Synaptic transmission

The transmitter at the neuromuscular junction is acetylcholine (ACh) which is packaged in vesicles in the presynaptic terminals. The arrival of an action potential in the presynaptic terminal causes a transient increase in the permeability of the terminal membrane to Ca^{2+} which in turn precipitates the simultaneous liberation of ACh from a number of vesicles. ACh diffuses across the narrow synaptic cleft, which is about 150 Å in width, and combines with receptors on the postsynaptic membrane. The postsynaptic receptors are only located in the immediate subsynaptic area in normal muscles and activation by ACh gives rise to local increases in ionic conductances, which generate the non-propogating, electrotonically decrementing end plate potentials (e.p.p.'s).

In muscle fibres which are focally innervated, the e.p.p. gives rise to a propagated muscle action potential which in turn invades the transverse tubular system, there to produce a translocation of Ca^{2+} which activates the contractile mechanism to produce single all-or-nothing twitches of the muscle at low frequencies of stimulation or, at higher frequencies of 30–100 Hz the single twitches fuse to produce a tetanic contraction, due to incomplete relaxation of the sliding filaments between each activation. The transmitter in multiple innervated muscles is related at a number of junctions and at each junction it produces an e.p.p. but these do not usually give rise to action potentials. Instead, the e.p.p.'s summate to produce slow graded depolarisations which evoke slow and graded contractures of the muscle fibres.

After dissociation of the ACh–receptor complex, the ACh is hydrolysed by the enzyme acetylcholinesterase which is located postsynaptically in the postjunctional folds. The choline is either removed in the circulation or else taken up again by an active transport process into the presynaptic terminals, where it is the precursor for ACh synthesised by the enzyme choline-acetyl-transferase.

In the absence of electrical activity in the motoneuronal axon, the ACh content of individual vesicles is released continuously in a random fashion. The contents of each vesicle produces unit, quantal changes in the potential across the postsynaptic membrane, termed miniature end plate potentials (m.e.p.p.'s) ranging in size from about 0.1 to 0.7 mV, due to random liberation of either single or multiple quanta of transmitter. The m.e.p.p.'s, like the e.p.p.'s, can be recorded with intracellular microelectrodes inserted into the postsynaptic cell close to the junctional region. Due to electrotonic decay, m.e.p.p.'s cannot be recorded if the electrode is moved far from the junction. Each quantum probably represents the contents of a single vesicle containing about 10 000 to 50 000 molecules of ACh. When a nerve impulse arrives in the terminal there is a sudden release of ACh from about 100 to 200 vesicles causing a large e.p.p. to occur after about 0.5 ms delay. The synaptic delay is made up of a short period required for the diffusion of ACh across the cleft (about 0.15 ms) and a somewhat longer period required for the release process.

Activation of the acetylcholine receptor

Peripheral receptors for ACh fall into two types both of which have been isolated by biochemical techniques. Muscarinic receptors are activated by ACh itself, by some choline esters such as acetyl-β-methylcholine and by muscarine. They are blocked by atropine. Muscarinic receptors are found in effector organs innervated by postganglionic parasympathetic fibres, e.g. in the heart and intestine. They are also found in autonomic ganglia (Chapter 3) and at a few sites innervated by postganglionic cholinergic sympathetic fibres, e.g. sweat glands. Nicotinic receptors are found at the neuromuscular junction and in autonomic ganglia. They are activated by ACh and by nicotine and are blocked competitively by either hexamethonium (autonomic ganglia) or by some curare-like substances (neuromuscular junction and ganglia). It will be evident that there are some differences between the nicotinic receptors in ganglia and at the neuromuscular junction. This is further exemplified by the fact that the ganglionic receptors are selectively activated by dimethylphenylpiperazinium whereas the receptors at the neuromuscular junction are selectively activated by phenyltrimethylammonium.

The interaction of a molecule of ACh with the receptor causes an increase in the cationic permeability of the postsynaptic membrane, especially to Na^+ and K^+, with a size limit not greater than twice the size of the hydrated K^+ ion. The influx of Na^+ causes a depolarisation of the membrane. The amplitude of the depolarisation depends on mass action kinetics and is therefore determined by the number of ACh molecules available for interaction. Since release from the nerve terminals is quantal in nature, the smallest m.e.p.p. observed corresponds to the activation by the content of one vesicle, containing 10 000–50 000 molecules of ACh.

Katz and Miledi determined by statistical techniques the amplitude of the elemental depolarisation caused by the interaction of a small number of molecules, one if the interaction is unimolecular, of ACh with the receptor. This elemental 'shot-effect' has an amplitude of about 0.3 μV and decays with a time constant of about 10 ms. The amplitude of the elemental shot-effect a is given by the expression:

$$a = \frac{2\bar{E}^2}{V} \text{mV},$$

where $\bar{E}^2$ is the variance of the membrane potential about the mean value produced by the external application of acetylcholine causing a mean depolarization of V mV.

Table 2.1. *Membrane noise and depolarisers of the neuromuscular junction (frog sartorius)*

	$a\ (\mu V)$	r (ms)
ACh	0.3	1.0
Carbachol	0.1	0.3–0.4
Suberyldicholine	0.4	1.65
Acetylthiocholine	0.08	0.12
Decamethonium	0.05	0.1

After Katz & Miledi (1973).
a is the elemental shot-effect; r is the duration of the opening of the ionic gate.

Since a is an elemental effect, the theory predicts that the value of a will be independent of the concentration of ACh administered or the resulting degree of depolarisation. This prediction has been substantiated experimentally.

A consideration of the data in Table 2.1 shows that the elemental effect differs in amplitude and time course with different depolarising agents.

Carbachol has a smaller elemental effect and a shorter duration of effect on the ionic gate than ACh but nevertheless is more potent in terms of affinity constants in depolarising the membrane. This can be explained on the basis that, unlike ACh, carbachol is not hydrolysed by acetylcholinesterase and molecules may therefore be available to interact repetitively with the receptors.

One possible explanation of the apparent variations in the values of a is that the different drugs open the same ionic gates but that the kinetics differ for each drug. However, other workers have measured the current rather than the voltage noise for different drugs and have shown that although there is a two-fold variation in the elemental conductance change (from 12.8 to 25 $p\Omega^{-1}$) there is a seven-fold variation in the duration of the opening times of the conductances, ranging from 0.83 to 5.6 ms. Thus there is not a simple linear relationship between the time for which the ionic gate is open and the amplitude of the elemental effect and it has been concluded that the channels may exist in different conformations, i.e. that there are different types of channel having different maximum conductances or, alternatively, that all channels have the same conformation but that different drugs may have different effects on local field strength, limiting access of ions to the channels. Magelby and Stevens have evidence that there are only two states for the channels, open or closed, and that each has its own rate constant.

It has been estimated that during the 1 ms for which the channel stays open with ACh, about 50 000 ions pass through, carrying a charge of about 7.5×10^{-5} C.

Neher and Sakmann have developed the technique still further so that they can measure the individual channel properties by direct measurement rather than indirectly by noise analysis. They have obtained data which are compatible with the earlier evidence and have also confirmed that the open times for the extrajunctional receptors in denervated, hypersensitive muscle are longer than those at the end plate.

SITES OF DRUG ACTION AT THE NEUROMUSCULAR JUNCTION

Drugs affecting neuromuscular transmission may act at one or more of three possible sites:

(*a*) On axonal conduction of the impulse into the nerve terminal.
(*b*) On presynaptic terminals, affecting transmitter storage, release or synthesis.
(*c*) On the postjunctional cell, either on the end plate or on the contractile mechanism at some step beyond the end plate.

Prejunctional drug action

Conduction. In addition to local anaesthetics, which non-selectively reduce excitability in all excitable tissues and so block axonal conduction of the nerve impulse as well as conduction of the impulse into the terminal, other drugs may affect electrical events in nerve terminals.

Cholinesterase inhibitors and in particular, neostigmine cause repetitive firing in the terminal on arrival of a single impulse down the axon. Normally, of course, a single axonal impulse would generate only a single action potential in the terminal. The depolarisation of the terminal may be so intense as to cause antidromic impulses to propagate up the axon. The mechanism of this effect is obscure but it does not seem to be related to the ability to inhibit acetylcholinesterase. Nevertheless, it may contribute to the effectiveness of neostigmine in treating patients with myasthenia gravis, although postsynaptic inhibition of cholinesterase is undoubtedly of major importance.

Veratrum alkaloids, e.g. germine monoacetate, are also of value in the treatment of myasthenia gravis and are known to cause repetitive firing not only in the nerve terminal but also in the muscle fibres themselves, which may be more important for the therapeutic effect.

The veratrum alkaloids do not change the sensitivity of the muscle to ACh nor do they change the frequency of m.e.p.p.'s or the amplitude of e.p.p.'s in doses which cause repetitive firing in frog muscle, although there may be a slight increase in m.e.p.p.'s in rat diaphragm muscle.

It seems likely that the action of the veratrum alkaloids on the terminals and on the muscle fibre membrane is due to a delayed closure of the Na^+ channels, although they probably also have other effects.

Tetrodotoxin blocks neuromuscular transmission by blocking Na^+ channels in all excitable membranes, including those of the presynaptic terminals and of the muscle fibres, so preventing the initiation of action potentials.

Synthesis of transmitter. A number of drugs can prevent the synthesis of ACh by blocking the enzyme choline acetyltransferase. However, they are not very specific and may also block acetylcholinesterase. Drugs of this type include diphenylbutylacetate and a number of styrylpyridine analogues. The most potent of the analogues is hexamethylene-1,4-(1-naphthylvinyl)-pyridinium-6-trimethyl ammonium, but this is almost as effective against acetylcholinesterase as it is against choline acetyltransferase *in vitro*.

In vivo, these substances block neuromuscular transmission but the blockade is probably related to a direct effect on the contractile mechanism rather than to an inhibition of choline acetyltransferase.

Inhibition of choline uptake. Hemicholinium (HC-3) is a quaternary ammonium drug which prevents the synthesis of ACh by blocking the uptake of the precursor, choline, into the terminal. In the first experiments with this substance, it was noted that when injected intravenously in rabbits it caused a respiratory paralysis and muscular relaxation which was aggravated by exercise. It was erroneously thought that this action was due to an effect on the brain stem, even though as a quaternary compound it was unlikely to cross the blood–brain barrier.

Since synthesis of ACh is only rate limiting for transmission in normal muscles at high rates of stimulation, HC-3 has little effect on the contractions of a muscle excited through its nerve at low rates of stimulation but there is a marked decline in the evoked twitches if the rate of stimulation is increased and the reduction can be counteracted by the administration of choline. This indicates that HC-3 blocks transmission by competing with choline for uptake sites on the terminal membrane. In confirmation of such a presynaptic site of action it has been shown that m.e.p.p.'s as well as e.p.p.'s are reduced by HC-3 and that the output of ACh, as measured directly by assay, is attenuated.

At high doses, HC-3 may also have a postjunctional curare-like effect.

Triethylcholine is transported almost as readily as choline and blocks neuromuscular transmission in a manner similar to that of HC-3. An earlier suggestion that triethylcholine might be acetylated, stored and released as a false transmitter, is of historical interest only as the first occasion on which this concept was invoked, but is no longer valid because attempts to isolate the acetylated derivative have not met with much success.

Tetraethylammonium (TEA) also has an action like that of

triethylcholine, but is better known for its ability to block K^+ channels. It may also have postsynaptic blocking action, especially pronounced in autonomic ganglia.

Storage of acetylcholine. A number of venoms are known to prevent the storage of ACh in the presynaptic vesicles.

In frog muscle, black widow spider venom causes at first a great increase in the number of m.e.p.p.'s recorded with an intracellular electrode and this is followed by a decrease in transmitter output and a block of neuromuscular transmission. It has been shown by electron microscopy that the terminals have lost their vesicles at this stage. In cats, similar effects are followed by a complete disintegration of the terminals.

β-bungarotoxin, obtained from the venom of the Formosan snake, and not to be confused with α-bungarotoxin which has a postsynaptic site of action, also has an action like that of the black widow spider venom on the presynaptic storage of ACh.

Mobilisation of transmitter. Not all of the ACh in the nerve terminal is immediately available for release, needing first to be 'mobilised'. Mobilisation, which may involve the movement of vesicles up to the release site on the membrane, is frequency dependent, is increased by an increase in extracellular Ca^{2+} in the medium or by depolarisation of the terminals with potassium chloride.

Some *antibiotics*, including neomycin, streptomycin and kanamycin, occasionally cause muscle weakness in therapy, and it has been suggested that they act by reducing transmitter mobilisation because they decrease the quantal content of the e.p.p.

Release of ACh. A highly toxic substance with a molecular weight of about 60 000 is produced by the anaerobic bacterium *Clostridium botulinum*. Botulinus toxin produces neuromuscular paralysis by virtue of the fact that it very effectively prevents the liberation of ACh from terminals without destroying the vesicles. It therefore acts upon the release process.

The fatal dose of toxin for a mouse is about 2×10^{-10} g/kg.

Making the assumption that a mouse has about 10^6 muscle fibres, Burgen has estimated that a fatal dose represents a concentration of the toxin corresponding to only forty molecules at each nerve ending. Even though the toxin is poorly absorbed from the gastrointestinal tract, the high potency is sufficient to ensure that it is absorbed in toxic amounts after ingestion.

The toxic effects of botulinus toxin are attributable to a paralysis of cholinergic systems throughout the body. They therefore include effects on the neuromuscular junction, at autonomic ganglia and at autonomic postganglionic cholinergic terminals. The symptoms include paralysis of eye muscles, causing diplopia, ptosis, dilated pupils and an inability to accommodate. Later, there is muscle weakness, respiratory distress, difficulty in swallowing and speaking, constipation and urinary retention.

It has been shown that the toxin does not affect the sensitivity of the postsynaptic membrane to ACh. There is no effect on the arrival of the impulse in the terminal nor is there any effect on the quantal size of the m.e.p.p. However, the frequency of spontaneous m.e.p.p.'s is greatly reduced and stimulation of the motor nerve elicits only a small or no e.p.p. and the assayed output of ACh is greatly reduced.

Simpson has suggested that the action of the toxin is dependent on ACh release. The block of transmission is prevented by maintaining a low concentration of Ca^{2+} in the medium to block ACh release, or by a maintained depolarisation of the terminals. It may be that there is a two-stage process, the first being a binding of the toxin to some unspecified membrane component, followed by interaction with a site exposed after release of ACh. It may be that the toxin acts by impairing Ca^{2+} entry. This explanation is supported by evidence (Lundh et al., 1976) that neuromuscular transmission in poisoned muscle may be alleviated by the use of Ca^{2+} ionophores, which carry Ca^{2+} across the membrane, or by tetraethylammonium (TEA), which prolongs the action potential by blocking K^+ channels, and so increases Ca^{2+} entry.

Guanidine sometimes alleviates muscle weakness in myasthenia. It increases e.p.p. amplitude but there is no change in the size or frequency of m.e.p.p.'s. There is no effect on the post-junctional sensitivity to ACh or on resting membrane potential or resistance. The effect is Ca^{2+}-dependent and it seems likely that it increases the ability of nerve impulses to release ACh from the presynaptic terminal.

Postjunctional drug action

Drugs causing a block of neuromuscular transmission are used as adjuvants in surgery to achieve good muscle relaxation, e.g. for abdominal surgery, or to prevent severe convulsions, such as those occurring in tetanus, or those produced by electroconvulsive therapy (ECT) in the treatment of psychiatric disorders.

A list of some of the more important neuromuscular block-ing drugs, together with some distinguishing pharmacological characteristics, is given in Fig. 2.2.

d-tubocurarine (d-TC) is a synthetic drug which is the active principle of the South American Indian arrow poison. In addition to blocking the nicotinic receptors at the neuromuscular junction it also blocks those in autonomic ganglia, resulting in a fall in blood pressure, decreased tone and motility of the gastrointestinal tract and a block of vagal effects. Histamine release is another important property which can lead to hypotension, bronchospasm and an increased bronchial and salivary secretion in man. These effects may be reduced by the administration of antihistamines.

The search for alternative drugs has concentrated on a reduction of these undesirable side-effects, together with different durations of action.

Gallamine is a short-acting, purely synthetic drug with a minimal effect on ganglia but it does reduce vagal effects by a mechanism that is not entirely clear and this may lead to tachycardia. *Pancuronium*, a synthetic steroidal neuromuscular blocking drug, is more potent than d-tubocurarine and has a similar duration of action but does not block ganglia or release histamine. The new substance (AH 8165) belonging to the azo-bis-aryl-imidazopyridium series has an action which is rapid in onset and brief in duration with minimal effects on the cardiovascular system.

Presynaptic   neostigmine   germine
Repetitive activation:

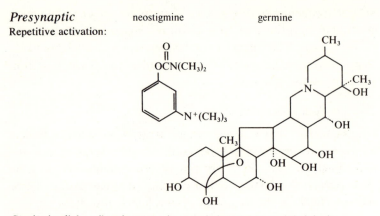

Synthesis: diphenylbutyl acetate, hexamethylene-1,4-(1-naphthylvinyl)-
pyridinium-6-trimethylammonium

Uptake: hemicholinium (HC-3)

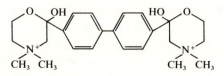

Storage: black widow spider venom, β-bungarotoxin
Mobilisation: neomycin, streptomycin
Release: botulinus toxin

Postsynaptic
Cholinesterase inhibitors:

                neostigmine   edrophonium

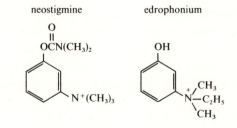

Fig. 2.2. Drugs affecting neuromuscular transmission.

Competitive blocking agents (reversible):

d-tubocurarine (d-TC)

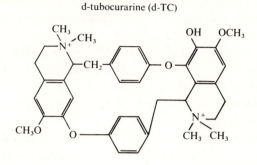

gallamine

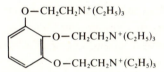

pancuronium

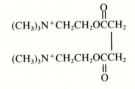

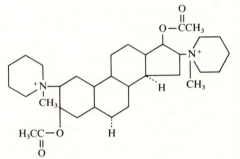

Competitive blocking agents (non-reversible): α-bungarotoxin

Desensitising blocking agents:

decamethonium

$(CH_3)_3N^+(CH_2)_{10}N^+(CH_3)_3$

succinylcholine

$(CH_3)_3N^+CH_2CH_2O\overset{\displaystyle O}{\overset{\|}{C}}CH_2$

$(CH_3)_3N^+CH_2CH_2O\underset{\displaystyle O}{\overset{\|}{C}}CH_2$

Metaphilic antagonists (reversible): dinaphthyl decamethonium (DNC-10).

Metaphilic antagonists (non-reversible): DNC-10 mustard

Fig. 2.2 (*cont.*)

The differential ability of some of these drugs to block the nicotinic receptors at the neuromuscular junction but not those in ganglia re-emphasise the point made earlier that the nicotinic receptors at the two sites are not identical.

All of the drugs so far mentioned act as competitive antagonists to ACh at the receptor sites. Another group of drugs, typified by *decamethonium* (C10) and *succinylcholine*, do not act as competitive antagonists and are referred to as depolarising or desensitising agents.

A characteristic of the depolarising agents is that they produce an initial muscle fasciculation before the onset of neuromuscular blockade. This may result in muscle pain postoperatively. C10 has minimal effects on ganglia or on histamine release and therefore has minimal effects on the circulation. Succinylcholine has a very brief duration of action due to the fact that it is a good substrate for plasma cholinesterase. However, in some patients with very low plasma cholinesterase it may have very prolonged effects in the normal dosage. These agents depolarise not only muscle but also autonomic ganglia. This action of succinylcholine on vagal ganglia may be sufficiently intense to cause bradycardia and hypotension. *Hexafluorenium* has a mild neuromuscular blocking action and in addition inactivates plasma cholinesterase. It is therefore used to prolong the action of succinylcholine.

Benzoquinonium has characteristics of both the competitive and the depolarising blocking drugs and in addition is a cholinesterase inhibitor.

α-bungarotoxin is not a clinically useful drug but it has been of great importance experimentally for the isolation of nicotinic receptors because it competes with ACh for the nicotinic receptor to form an irreversible drug–receptor complex.

Mechanism of neuromuscular blockade by competitive receptor antagonists. The theory of drug–receptor interaction based upon the law of mass action predicts that in the presence of a reversible, competitive antagonist the log dose–response curve for an agonist will be shifted to the right and that the curve will remain parallel to the control curve obtained in the absence of the antagonist and that the maximum response obtained from the tissue will remain unchanged. Curare-like drugs should therefore be expected to conform to these criteria since they are believed to be competitive, reversible antagonists of ACh at the nicotinic receptors at the motor end plate.

Dose–response curves for ACh are easily obtained upon the frog rectus muscle preparation. At low concentrations of d-tubo-curarine producing dose ratios for the agonist (ACh) of about 100 the curves remain reasonably parallel and the maximum response does not change appreciably. Thus, at these concentrations of antagonist there seems to be a competitive interaction. At higher concentrations there is a progressive departure from parallelism and the maximum response declines. On the frog sartorius muscle in which Jenkinson compared the depolarisation of the end plate produced by carbachol in the presence and absence of d-tubocurarine, the departure from parallelism and the reduction of the maximum response was even more marked at relatively low concentrations of the antagonist. In the tibialis muscle of the cat, Paton and Waud showed that gallamine caused very marked discrepancies from the anticipated curves.

These results are difficult to explain simply in terms of competitive antagonism but it has been suggested by Paton and Waud that the responses to the agonists may not be equilibrium responses and that the antagonists in some way change the equilibria. Thus, a dose–response curve in this instance does not give unequivocal support for the competitive nature of the anticholinergic action of d-tubocurarine or gallamine.

Convincing evidence showing that the interaction of d-tubo-curarine with acetylcholine at the motor end plate is competitive has been obtained by Katz and Miledi in their experiments on membrane noise. They predicted that if the antagonism was truly competitive in nature, then the amplitude of the elemental shot-effect produced by the interaction of one molecule of ACh with the receptor should be unaffected by the presence of the antagonist. They have found that neither d-tubocurarine nor the irreversible antagonist α-bungarotoxin changes the amplitude of the ACh shot-effect, a.

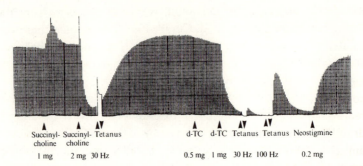

Fig. 2.3. Contractions of the tibialis muscle of a cat anaesthetised with chloralose to electrical stimulation of peripheral stump of the sciatic nerve every 5 s. The record shows that an intravenous injection of 1 mg of succinylcholine caused a facilitation of the contractions, whereas a larger dose caused only a transient facilitation followed by block of transmission during which tetanic stimulation at 30 Hz caused a small but maintained contraction. D-tubocurarine (0.5 and 1 mg) caused only a block of transmission, during which a tetanus (100 Hz) was not maintained but gave rise to post-tetanic potentiation. Neostigmine (0.2 mg) reversed the blockade of neuromuscular transmission.

From time to time it is suggested that although curare-like drugs undoubtedly have a postsynaptic blocking action on the ACh receptors, the most important action for neuromuscular blockade may be produced by an effect on the presynaptic terminal. This theory is not generally accepted and is mainly based upon the results of electrophysiological experiments on postsynaptic potentials. Perhaps the strongest evidence against this view is the observation that when the amount of ACh released from the presynaptic terminals is assayed directly, rather than by inference from the electrophysiological changes, there is no change when neuromuscular transmission is blocked by d-tubocurarine.

Mechanism of neuromuscular block by decamethonium and succinylcholine. In contrast to the relatively clear-cut mode of action of the curare-like drugs, the mechanism by which the depolarising drugs decamethonium and succinylcholine block neuromuscular transmission is more complex and not so well established.

The systemic administration of decamethonium or succinylcholine causes in mammals a muscle fasciculation which is relatively short-lived (Fig. 2.3). During this phase of the effect, the muscle twitches elicited by nerve stimulation may at first be enhanced but are later reduced and ultimately completely blocked. The fasciculation is a reasonably clear indication that the muscle membrane has been depolarised in some way by the drug. The conclusion is supported by experiments on the multiple innervated rectus abdominis muscle of the frog on which the depolarising drugs cause a sustained contracture and depolarisation which is antagonised, like that of ACh, by d-tubocurarine. Some early experiments of Burns and Paton in 1951 seemed to support the idea that the blockade of neuromuscular transmission was due to an excessive depolarisation of the postsynaptic membrane which inactivates the Na^+ carrier, so preventing the production of propagated action potentials. In these experiments on the gracilis muscle of the cat there was a similarity in the time-course of muscle depolarisation and the blockade of transmission by decamethonium.

However, the close correspondence between depolarisation and block seen on the gracilis muscle of the cat is not found in a variety of other test situations (Fig. 2.4). Even in the early work on mammalian muscles it was realised that different muscles in the cat showed different responses to decamethonium, and that there were species differences. In all muscles of the monkey, dog, rabbit and rat and in the soleus muscle of the cat it was thought that decamethonium and succinylcholine produced a 'dual' block, changing with time from a depolarising type of blockade to a non-depolarising type. However, in the tibialis and gracilis muscles of the cat and probably in man the type of block produced was thought to be due to depolarisation of the end plate.

It is difficult to understand on kinetic grounds how a drug could change its mechanism of action with time on a given tissue from an initial depolarising mechanism of blockade to a subsequent non-depolarizing, competitive type of antagonism. An alternative theory based upon the concept of receptor desensitisation originally developed by Katz and Thesleff and subsequently considerably expanded by Rang and Ritter to include the concept of metaphilic antagonism offers a more attractive explanation based upon dynamic changes in receptor conformation produced

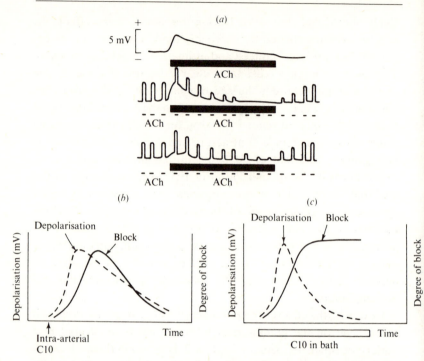

Fig. 2.4. Desensitisation, depolarisation and neuromuscular block. (*a*) Iontophoresis of ACh on frog muscle. A prolonged (15 s) administration of ACh causes a depolarisation which is not sustained, and the effect of repeated small administrations of ACh is reduced by the prolonged administration, even when the depolarisation produced initially is minute. After Katz, B. and Thesleff, S. (1967) *J. Physiol.*, **138**, 63. (*b*) The intra-arterial injection of C10 in a cat (gracilis muscle) causes a block of neuromuscular transmission and a depolarisation of the muscle with a somewhat different time-course. After Burns, B. D. and Paton, W. D. (1951) *J. Physiol.*, **115**, 41. (*c*) Bath application of C10 to frog muscle. The addition of decamethonium to Ringer's solution in the bath causes a sustained block of neuromuscular transmission but only a transient depolarisation. After Thesleff, S. (1955) *Acta Physiol. Scand.*, **34**, 218.

by the action of substances such as decamethonium and succinylcholine.

Desensitisation and metaphilic antagonism. Katz and Thesleff showed that a number of depolarising agents including ACh, nicotine, decamethonium and succinylcholine produced a short-lived depolarisation of the frog sartorius muscle and a block of

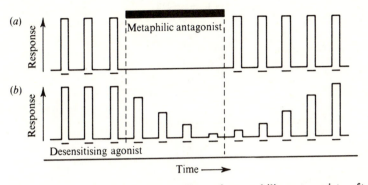

Fig. 2.5. (a) Lack of apparent effect of metaphilic antagonists after washout when desensitising agonist is not administered during administration of antagonist, contrasted with marked effect when both are present together (b).

synaptic transmission which reached a maximum after the depolarisation had subsided (Fig. 2.4). The block persisted, in the absence of depolarisation, for as long as the agent was present in the bath fluid. They also showed that the microelectrophoretic application of ACh to the end plate region in amounts sufficient to cause only a very small and waning depolarisation were sufficient, if continued for a long enough period, to block the action of short pulses of ACh which were also applied microelectrophoretically. Such small depolarisations by ACh are not adequate to cause an inactivation of the sodium carrier mechanism and it was thought that prolonged exposure of the receptors to ACh had in some way decreased their sensitivity, i.e. had desensitised them to the transmitter.

Rang and Ritter found that the dinaphthyl derivative of decamethonium, DNC-10 only blocked the action of cholinergic agonists on frog and chick muscle if the muscle had been previously exposed to the agonist (Fig. 2.5). The rate of onset of the antagonism was faster if the agonist was given at frequent intervals and was slower with more dispersed application. The block was greater with some agonists than with others. For example, the blocking action with DNC-10 was greater when decamethylene-bis-trimethylammonium (C10-TMA) was used as the agonist than it was with C10 or carbachol. This was due to

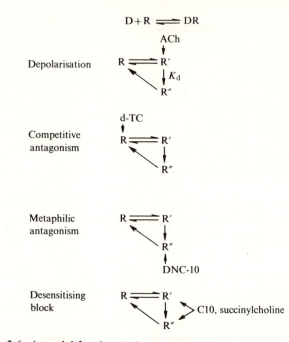

Fig. 2.6. A model for depolarisation, desensitisation and block.

the fact that C10-TMA produces more desensitisation than the other drugs. This special type of drug antagonism by DNC-10 was termed 'metaphilic' antagonism, and it depends on the presence of a desensitising agent.

The slightly modified scheme in Fig. 2.6 shows a theoretical basis for the actions of competitive antagonists of the curare type, of desensitising, depolarising blocking agents of the C10 type and of the metaphilic antagonists like DNC-10.

An agonist or antagonist, D, combines with the receptor R to form the drug–receptor complex DR. If the drug is an agonist then it will have affinity for the receptor conformation R', an isomer of R. The conformation R' is that form which opens the ionic channels in the membrane to allow the entry of sodium ions which cause depolarisation. The amount of depolarisation depends upon the affinity of the drug for R'. In the extreme case when D has a high affinity for R but not for R' the drug will represent an agent showing pure competitive antagonism against the transmitter ACh.

If the drug has affinity for R' and R", it will cause some initial depolarisation but in the continued presence of D there will be a slow conversion of $_1$DR' to DR" at a rate determined by the desensitisation rate constant K_d. If the recovery rate constant is also slow, then there will be a slow net accumulation of R". There will then be less available R' for combination with D to form DR' and so the depolarisation will diminish, as seen with C10 on many tissues. The effectiveness of the natural transmitter ACh will also diminish resulting in a blockade of neuromuscular transmission.

It may therefore be predicted that C10 should produce a conductance change which should decline with time. This has been substantiated in experiments with microelectrophoretic administration of C10 and in other experiments in which high concentrations of C10 were administered to the medium bathing isolated rat diaphragm muscle. In the latter experiments it was also found that the recovery of the membrane potential after carbachol or low concentrations of C10, normally occurring within a few minutes, despite continued application, could be prevented by treatment with ouabain. This indicates that activation of the sodium pump mechanism may be partially responsible for the recovery of the membrane potential in the continued presence of the agonist. Such a mechanism may supplement the desensitisation, which is unaffected by ouabain.

The difference between neuromuscular blocking agents of the competitive type and those of the desensitising type is therefore seen to lie, in terms of the theory outlined above, in their differing affinities for R and R" and possibly, in part, to the ability of the latter to activate the sodium pump by some as yet unknown mechanism.

The metaphilic antagonists have a selective affinity for R" and no affinity for R. They therefore rely for their antagonism on the production of R" by a desensitising agent.

In summary, the neuromuscular blockade produced by desensitising agents such as C10 or succinylcholine may be attributed to the production of a desensitised conformation of the receptor, together with possibly some activation of the sodium pump, both of which will cause a reduction in the size of e.p.p.'s and reduce the efficacy of synaptic transmission. The initial depolarisation causes muscle contractions. However, only at extremely high levels of depolarisation in some muscles is there likely to be an inactivation of the sodium carrier and it appears unnecessary to invoke this mechanism to explain the block of neuromuscular transmission.

Characterisation of neuromuscular blocking agents. Neuromuscular blocking agents which act competitively, e.g. d-tubocurarine (d-TC) can be distinguished from those which cause depolarisation, e.g. C10 by a number of tests in whole animals or on isolated tissues. The differences seen are presumed to be due to their differing modes of action, although the precise explanation is not always clear.

(1) A muscle depolarisation is absent with competitive antagonists. They therefore do not cause initial muscle fasciculation when injected intravenously in mammals nor do they cause a contracture of multiple innervated frog muscle. In birds, which have both focally and multiple innervated muscle fibres, they cause a muscle paralysis of a flaccid type, in contrast to the depolarising agents which cause spastic paralysis characterised by opisthotonus and rigid limb extension.

(2) Cholinesterase inhibitors, e.g. neostigmine, reverse block by d-TC but not by C10, due to an improvement in the safety factor for transmission.

(3) Tetanic stimulation of the motor nerve to mammalian muscle causes a maintained contraction of the muscle due to incomplete relaxation of the contractile elements between each stimulus. After administration of d-TC this tetanic contraction is no longer maintained. The effect is not evident during the early stages of blockade by C10. The decline in tetanic muscle tension after d-TC can be attributed to a progressive reduction in the amount of ACh liberated with each stimulus, i.e. transmitter depletion. The e.p.p.'s then become smaller until they are finally unable to elicit a muscle action potential. In untreated muscle

the e.p.p. does not fall below the threshold for the initiation of propagated muscle action potentials because there there is a high safety factor for transmission, i.e. the degree of receptor activation by ACh is far greater than that required to produce an e.p.p. which is just adequate to initiate an action potential. In curarised muscle a proportion of the receptors are blocked and the safety factor for transmission is therefore reduced and transmission fails during transmitter depletion.

(4) Post-tetanic potentiation (PTP) of the twitches is evident after block of transmission by d-TC but not after C10. PTP is attributed to the increased entry of Ca^{2+} per unit time at tetanic frequencies of stimulation, leading to an increased transmitter output per stimulus. This is not evident during tetanisation because of the opposing depletion of transmitter, but becomes evident when a low rate of stimulation is resumed, presumably because the equilibrium state is restored only after tetanisation. PTP is not readiy observed in noncurarised muscles because the safety factor ensures that every muscle fibre contracts with every stimulus and further post-tetanic increases in ACh output can have no additional effect.

Denervation hypersensitivity

Muscles which have been denervated by cutting the motor nerve supply and allowing sufficient time for the nerve fibres distal to the cut to degenerate become hypersensitive to ACh. The hypersensitivity is due to a spread of receptors along the muscle fibres, although the original end plate region continues to be the most sensitive part of the membrane. Similar effects may be produced by irreversibly blocking the postjunctional receptors with α-bungarotoxin.

The hypersensitivity and the receptor dispersion may be counteracted by direct electrical stimulation of the muscle fibres, showing that the control of the receptors is partly a function of muscle activity. However, the possibility that there may be 'trophic' factors liberated from the nerve terminals which prevent the spread of receptor sites has not been eliminated.

The characteristics of the new extrajunctional receptors on

denervated muscle are not identical with those of the receptors normally found only at the end plate. Although both are nicotinic in type, the hypersensitivity which also develops to d-tubocurarine is not as great as for ACh, and, for a particular agonist, the channel open times are longer at extrajunctional than at end plate regions.

Myasthenia gravis

About 1 in every 6000 persons is afflicted with a crippling disease of the neuromuscular junction called myasthenia gravis. The disease strikes either suddenly or gradually and usually appears between the ages of 10 and 40 years. The incidence is greater in women than in men but the distribution of the disease is unaffected by geography, race or climate. It seems very likely that myasthenia is an autoimmune disease. Electronmicroscopic studies have shown that it is accompanied by marked changes in the innervation of the muscle fibres, including a reduction in the number and size of the nerve terminals and an increase in the diameter of the synaptic cleft. It is these anatomical changes which no doubt account for the reduced size of the m.e.p.p.'s recorded electrophysiologically.

In part, the myasthenic symptoms are not dissimilar from those produced by neuromuscular blocking drugs like d-tubocurarine and myasthenic patients show a marked increase in sensitivity to competitive neuromuscular blocking drugs. The muscle weakness increases during repetitive muscle activity and decreases on resting. It tends to increase progressively throughout the day.

In about 10% of patients there is a thymoma and in many more there is a milder thymitis. Thymectomy improves the condition in a high proportion of myasthenics, although only about one-third are reported to have complete remission of symptoms.

About 30% of patients have circulating antibodies reacting with striated muscle and this has led to the testing of a number of immunosuppressive agents, usually without success. ACTH may have some ameliorative effect but it probably acts indirectly by an action on the thymus gland, rather than directly as an immunosuppressive agent.

Experimentally, a substance called 'thymin' has been isolated from the thymus of guinea pigs in which immunity has been produced and on injection into control animals this substance causes muscle weakness. However, the relevance of this finding to the clinical condition of myasthenia, although alluringly attractive, remains to be established.

Myasthenic symptoms may be reduced by the administration of a cholinesterase inhibitor. Neostigmine is generally used because it has a fairly long duration of action and does not pass the blood–brain barrier. Germine monoacetate has also found some followers. A very short-acting anticholinesterase, edrophonium, is used as a diagnostic test for myasthenia gravis.

Related conditions, such as myasthenic syndrome, are not improved by the cholinesterase inhibitors. In this condition the anatomical changes at the end plate are milder and differ from those occurring in myasthenia gravis. The quantal content of the e.p.p. is decreased and the response to a single stimulus to the motor nerve is attenuated. This suggests that the defect may be in the release mechanism for the synaptic transmitter.

CHAPTER THREE

Pharmacology of the autonomic nervous system

PHYSIOLOGICAL BASIS

The autonomic nervous system is an efferent system conveying impulses from the central nervous system to the periphery. It controls the activity of all bodily functions except those of the skeletal muscles which are controlled by the somato-motor system discussed in Chapter 2. It therefore affects such diverse functions as salivary secretion, sweating, movement and secretions of the gastrointestinal tract, the heart rate and the calibre of the blood vessels, the secretions of the pineal gland, the contraction of the urinary bladder and its internal sphincter, penile erection, adrenaline secretion by the adrenal glands, accommodation of the eye and the diameter of the pupil. Interference with the autonomic system by pharmacological means will therefore lead to widespread effects, limited only by the specificity of the drugs for particular synaptic sites.

There are two major divisions of the autonomic nervous system. The sympathetic division originates from preganglionic nerve cell bodies lying in the intermedio-lateral part of the grey matter of the spinal cord in the thoracic and upper lumbar regions. The parasympathetic division originates from nerve cells located in brain stem and intermedio-lateral regions of the sacral spinal cord. The preganglionic neurones give rise mainly to myelinated B fibres with a conduction velocity slower than that of the slowest motor axons innervating skeletal muscle but faster than those of the non-myelinated C fibres of the postganglionic nerves.

A comparison with the skeleto-motor system (Fig. 3.1) shows that a major distinguishing feature of the autonomic nervous system is the interposition of a peripheral ganglionic synapse between the cells of origin in the CNS and the peripheral organ which is innervated. In the sympathetic nervous system, the ganglion is situated either in the paravertebral chain ganglia or in

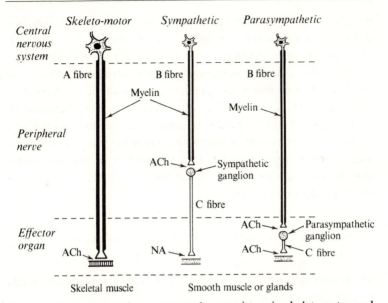

Fig. 3.1. Comparison of structure and transmitters in skeletomotor and autonomic nervous system.

one of the special sympathetic ganglia, such as the cervical sympathetic, stellate, coeliac, inferior mesenteric or hypogastric ganglia. This arrangement differs from that usually found in the parasympathetic system, where the ganglia are often embedded in the effector organ and give rise to only short postganglionic fibres; the ciliary ganglion, giving rise to postganglionic para-sympathetic nerves to the orbit, is an exception.

The most important transmitters in the autonomic nervous system are ACh and noradrenaline (NA). ACh is the transmitter liberated from the terminals of the preganglionic fibres in both the sympathetic and parasympathetic systems and causes excitation of the postganglionic neurones. ACh is also the transmitter at the endings of parasympathetic fibres on the effector organs where it may function either as an inhibitory transmitter, e.g. in slowing the heart, or as an excitatory transmitter, e.g. in causing contrac-tions of some of the smooth muscle in the alimentary tract and the urinary bladder. Noradrenaline is liberated from the postganglionic endings of sympathetic nerves and may also function either as an excitatory transmitter, e.g. increasing the heart rate, or as an inhibitory transmitter, e.g. inhibiting the movements of the intestine. The chromaffin cells of the adrenal medulla may be considered as modified postganglionic sympathetic ganglion cells which are able to synthesise adrenaline from noradrenaline by N-methylation and to liberate the amine into the circulation where it may exert effects as a hormone, rather than as a transmitter. Dopamine is also involved as a transmitter in the autonomic ganglia, although its precise role in the physiological operation of the ganglion remains elusive.

SITES OF DRUG ACTION IN THE AUTONOMIC NERVOUS SYSTEM

Drugs may act either at ganglionic sites or at peripheral adrenergic or cholinergic synapses.

Ganglionic synapses

It was originally believed that synaptic transmission in autonomic ganglia was relatively simple and involved only the liberation of ACh from the presynaptic nerve terminals with a simple post-synaptic excitation of the postganglionic neurones. Although this is undoubtedly the most important event in the function of the ganglion, it is now clear that there are other synaptic events, the practical consequences of which are not yet very certain.

The fact that ganglionic synapses are sensitive to nicotine was recognised by Langley at the turn of the century. He painted tinctures of nicotine on the courses of autonomic nerves and showed that only when the nicotine was applied to discrete points on the nerves, which we now know to be the ganglia, was any effect observed. At low concentrations of nicotine there was an effect which could be mimicked by stimulation of the sympathetic nerve whereas at higher concentrations there was first an excitant effect, similar to that at low concentrations, but this was followed by a failure of nerve stimulation to produce any effect. This dual excitatory and inhibitory action of nicotine is due to interaction of the agent with the postganglionic nicotinic receptors for ACh to cause depolarisation and excitation, followed by a blocking action due to desensitisation. This is similar to that seen with nicotine and other agents at the neuromuscular junction. Langley used this simple technique to map out the autonomic nervous system as we now know it.

The ganglionic nicotinic receptors are also activated by tetra-methylammonium, which has a relatively brief duration of action and by dimethylphenylpiperazinium (DMPP), which distinguishes the ganglionic receptors from those at the neuromuscular junction.

Ganglionic blocking agents. The cervical sympathetic nerve–nictitating membrane preparation of the anaesthetised cat is a relatively simple preparation which has been widely used to study the action of drugs on sympathetic ganglionic transmission. The nictitating membrane, or third eyelid of the cat is a mobile structure composed of smooth muscle which is innervated only by noradrenergic terminals of the postganglionic fibres originating from the superior cervical ganglion. The preganglionic cervical sympathetic nerve is a long nerve which courses together with the vagus in the neck and can easily be separated from the vagus by dissection. The postganglionic nerve is accessible for stimulation for only a few millimetres rostral to the ganglion. Drugs may be administered either systemically or by local arterial injection into the ganglion. The ganglion may also be perfused *in situ* and with such a technique it has been conclusively demonstrated that ACh is liberated from the ganglion during stimulation of the pre-ganglionic nerve.

Drugs which selectively block ganglionic transmission block the contractions of the nictitating membrane evoked by preganglionic nerve stimulation but not those evoked by postganglionic nerve stimulation. *Hexamethonium*, hexamethylene-bis (trimethylam-monium) is a drug which classically blocks ganglionic transmission by competitively interacting with ACh at the nicotinic receptors. Systemic administration therefore blocks the contractions of the membrane in response to either preganglionic nerve stimulation or to intra-arterially injected ACh, but does not affect the response to postganglionic stimulation or injected catecholamines.

Hexamethonium (Fig. 3.2) is one of a series of bisquaternary

Ganglionic blocking agents

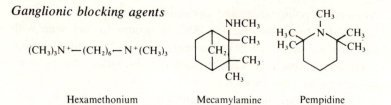

$(CH_3)_3N^+—(CH_2)_6—N^+(CH_3)_3$

Hexamethonium   Mecamylamine   Pempidine

Drugs affecting peripheral noradrenergic terminals

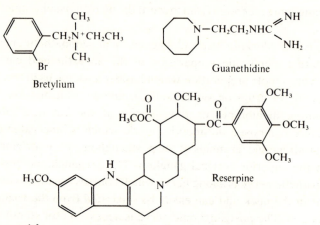

Bretylium

Guanethidine

Reserpine

Drugs with an uncertain mode of action (see text)

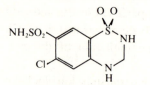

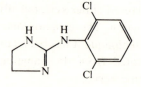

Hydrochlorothiazide   Clonidine

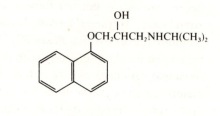

α-methyl DOPA   Propranolol

Fig. 3.2. Drugs which have been used in hypertension.

ammonium compounds synthesised in the 1940s in attempts to find drugs which could be of value as neuromuscular blocking agents. It will be recalled that longer-chain members of this series, in particular decamethonium, are effective in blocking transmission at the neuromuscular junction. However, the shorter-chain members of the series had ganglionic blocking activity, with maximum potency residing in hexamethonium, with six carbon atoms in the chain. At that time (1944–50) one of the treatments for high blood pressure (essential hypertension) was extirpation of the sympathetic chain, a somewhat drastic procedure. Ganglion blocking agents seemed to be a far preferable alternative. For a while, hexamethonium and, to a lesser extent pentolinium, were used with some success. Because these substances are quaternary compounds they are poorly absorbed from the gut, necessitating systemic administration for optimal effects. In this respect, pentolinium was slightly better than hexamethonium and had a longer duration of action.

A major disadvantage with ganglion blocking agents is that they block both sympathetic and parasympathetic ganglia, leading to a number of unpleasant side-effects including mydriasis, paralytic ileus, dryness of the mouth and eyes and difficulties with micturition.

Unsuccessful synthetic programmes were undertaken in attempts to find drugs which would have a preferential affinity for the nicotinic receptors in sympathetic ganglia.

The usefulness of the bisquaternary polymethylene compounds was short lived. In 1956 the secondary amine *mecamylamine* and in 1958 the cyclic nitrogen compound *pempidine* were introduced as orally-active ganglionic blocking agents. They had longer durations of action than the quaternary compounds but they act in the same way and so are accompanied by similar side-effects on the parasympathetic system. In addition, they penetrate the blood–brain barrier to some degree and so caused some unpleasant effects on the CNS. The reign of the non-quaternary ganglionic blocking agents was even briefer than that of the quaternary compounds because in 1959 they were superseded by the adrenergic neuronal blocking agents with a selective effect upon the sympathetic nervous system.

Hypertension. At the present time the treatment of essential hypertension includes not only the adrenergic neurone blocking agents (see below) but also drugs such as α-methyldopa and β-blocking agents which probably act in quite a different fashion. *Clonidine* is an antihypertensive drug which may act by an activation of α-adrenoceptors for noradrenaline in the CNS, or by activation of a presynaptic α-adrenoceptor to prevent noradrenaline release peripherally.

The treatment for high blood pressure over the years has been extremely varied and, although it is not a generally accepted point of view, Goldring has even questioned whether one is only treating a symptom which may have some compensatory beneficial effect on the renal and vascular changes which are not necessarily caused by the high blood pressure *per se.* He points out that treatment has ranged from protein or salt restriction, extract of garlic, methylene blue, watermelon seeds, vitamin A, thiocyanate, adrenalectomy, sympathectomy, prefrontal lobotomy, ganglion blockers and now the newer drugs. It is obvious that some of these remedies were used with little justification and they serve perhaps to illustrate our lack of real understanding of the basic problems. Nevertheless it is generally accepted that treatment of essential hypertension by modern drugs represents an acceptable and effective method of alleviating symptoms and thereby prolonging life.

d-tubocurarine, a neuromuscular blocking agent, also blocks the nicotinic receptors in ganglia. This is probably a partial explanation of the fall in blood pressure which accompanies the administration of this substance. Indeed, orthostatic hypotension is a major drawback to most antihypertensive agents which act by interfering with peripheral sympathetic function.

Ganglionic receptors. In 1961, Eccles and Libet studied electrical responses in partially curarised cervical sympathetic ganglia isolated from the rabbit. They demonstrated three major electrical components in the potentials recorded from the surface of the ganglion after preganglionic stimulation which have led subsequently to many investigations of their significance.

The first, negative wave (N-wave) of rather brief duration is caused by a postganglionic depolarisation resulting from activation of nicotinic receptors. The second positive wave (P-wave), is greatly increased by repetitive activation of the preganglionic nerve and is due to postganglionic hyperpolarisation and a late negative wave (LN-wave) is again due to depolarisation of the postganglionic neurone. Drug interactions indicate that the P-wave involves the activation of muscarinic receptors and that, in addition, the P-wave also involved catecholamine receptors. They concluded that the ganglion must contain an interneurone which is activated by ACh acting on muscarinic receptors and which liberates a catecholamine which hyperpolarises the postganglionic cell. The interneurone has now been identified as a 'small intensely fluorescent' interneurone which liberates dopamine as a transmitter. They further concluded that the postganglionic neurone was activated by ACh acting on both nicotinic and muscarinic receptors. These conclusions are summarised in Fig. 3.3.

It has now been demonstrated that sympathetic ganglia respond to injected ACh in a complex fashion which can be separated by the use of selective antagonists into nicotinic and muscarinic components.

Furthermore, postganglionic discharges are readily evoked by muscarinic receptor activators such as muscarine, acetyl-β-methylcholine and McNeill A-343, all of which are blocked by atropine. Rather surprisingly, the administration of anticholinesterases also gives a prolonged discharge which is blocked by atropine but not by hexamethonium.

Thus it is established that muscarinic receptors in ganglia can be activated by pharmacological means or by electrical stimulation of the preganglionic nerve, but their physiological function is obscure. There is some evidence that postganglionic discharges evoked reflexly or by electrical stimulation of the hypothalamus are only partially blocked by hexamethonium, but are effectively blocked by a combination of hexamethonium and atropine. This indicates that the muscarinic receptors may have some significance for the physiological operation of sympathetic ganglia.

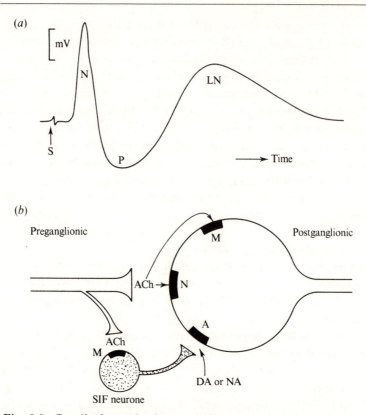

Fig. 3.3. Ganglionic mechanisms. (a) Diagrammatic representation of sequence of postganglionic potentials evoked by a stimulus (S) to the preganglionic nerve. N, surface-negative wave of depolarisation; P, surface-positive wave of hyperpolarisation; LN, late surface-negative wave of depolarisation. (b) Postulated ganglionic synapses causing the recorded wave form. N, nicotinic receptors (blocked by hexamethonium or d-tubocurarine); M, muscarinic receptors (blocked by atropine); A, adrenoceptor (blocked by dibenamine); SIF, small, intensely fluorescent neurone.

The physiological function of the dopaminergic interneurone is even more obscure, but there is evidence that dopamine acts via an increase in cyclic AMP. It is possible that a cyclic nucleotide (cyclic GMP) is also involved in the muscarinic actions of ACh in ganglia.

Yet another complication in ganglionic pharmacology is that

dopamine may act as a negative feedback transmitter upon the preganglionic cholinergic terminals.

Thus it may be seen that the ganglion, which some years ago appeared to be a simple relay station on sympathetic nerves, probably performs a number of highly complex, integrative and control functions which have yet to be completely understood. Although most studies have been concentrated upon sympathetic ganglia, recent studies have shown that events occurring in parasympathetic ganglia are rather similar.

Peripheral noradrenergic synapses

The pharmacology of peripheral noradrenergic synapses has been well documented in a number of excellent articles and books (see list of selected reading) and so will only be summarised here to complete our study of drug interactions at synapses.

Some of the concepts which have arisen from studies on peripheral noradrenergic synapses are particularly important because they have contributed a great deal to ideas concerning the actions of numerous drugs on the central nervous system, which we shall consider later.

Receptors. Noradrenaline liberated from postganglionic sympathetic nerves or adrenaline from the adrenal medulla may produce excitation or inhibition of effector organs by interaction with α- or β-adrenoceptors.

α-adrenoceptors are responsible for vasoconstriction and for contraction of some smooth muscles, e.g. the nictitating membrane or for relaxation of others, e.g. in the intestine. β_1-adrenoceptors are responsible for acceleration of the heart beat and an increase in the force of contraction (positive inotropic effect), whereas β_2-adrenoceptors cause vasodilatation and relaxation of respiratory smooth muscle.

Noradrenaline and adrenaline interact with all receptors, as might be expected, although there are differences in relative potencies on each type of receptor. β-adrenoceptors are selectively activated by isoprenaline whereas phenylethylamine has a relatively selective effect on α-adrenoceptors.

Antagonists at α-adrenoceptors include such substances as dibenamine, phenoxybenzamine and tolazoline. They are not of great therapeutic value and are of no value in treating hypertension unless caused by excessive levels of circulating catecholamines, as in phaeochomocytoma.

β-adrenoceptors are blocked non-selectively by dichloroisoprenaline and proprandol, but practolol has a relatively greater effect on β_1-adrenoceptors than on β_2-adrenoceptors. Salbutamol is a selective agonist for β_2-adrenoceptors, but no selective β_2-adrenoceptor antagonist is yet available, perhaps because there is no obvious therapeutic application for such a drug. Although butoxamine is an antagonist at β_2-adrenoceptors, it is also a partial agonist at β_1-adrenoceptors.

Activation of β_2-adrenoceptors in the bronchi by *isoprenaline* to cause muscle relaxation is used successfully to treat asthmatic bronchoconstriction. However, the stimulant effect on β_1-adrenoceptors in the heart is a complication which in overdosage has led to fatalities. *Salbutamol* is somewhat safer in this respect.

β-blocking agents, e.g. *propranolol*, have found use in some cardiac abnormalities as anti-arrhythmic drugs, but it is not certain that this property is directly related to the β-receptor blocking action because the effective drugs also have local anaesthetic properties. β-blockers are currently receiving considerable attention as a new class of antihypertensive agents, although the mechanism of action remains elusive. They are also effective in angina pectoris by reducing the work of the heart.

There is considerable clinical interest in developing agents which have selective effects upon β-adrenoceptors. For example, an agent which increases force of contraction of the heart, but not the rate, both of which appear to be related to β_1-adrenoceptors, would be useful in myocardial ischaemia: dobutamine shows some promise in this respect. Conversely a substance which decreased heart rate but not the force of contraction would also be extremely useful but no such agent is currently available. A good β_2 antagonist would be an aid in decreasing peripheral shunting in septic shock and salbutamol is a selective β_2 agonist which has applications as a bronchodilator.

β-adrenoceptor blocking agents are of value in angina pectoris and as anti-arrhythmic drugs and attempts have been made to find drugs with a selective effect upon β_1-adrenoceptors ('cardio-selective' β-blockers). A disadvantage with the non-selective β-blockers is that they may decrease blood flow in the ischaemic heart, so precipitating heart failure. This is probably due to an unmasking of α-adrenoceptors in the coronary circulation, causing vasoconstriction. However, practalol blocks only β_1-receptors and leaves the β_2 vasodilator mechanisms intact which can still counteract the α-mediated vasoconstriction. Thus practalol does not decrease blood flow in the ischaemic heart.

Effects on presynaptic terminals. Many drugs affect noradrenergic transmission by an action on presynaptic noradrenergic terminals. Noradrenaline is synthesised within terminals from the amino acid tyrosine which is first hydroxylated by the rate-limiting enzyme tyrosine hydroxylase to dihydroxyphenylalanine (DOPA). This is converted to dopamine by DOPA decarboxylase. Dopamine β-hydroxylase hydroxylates the β-carbon atom of the ethylamine side chain to yield noradrenaline. In the chromaffin cells of the adrenal medulla noradrenaline is N-methylated by phenyletha-nolamine-N-methyl transferase to yield adrenaline (Fig. 3.4).

Noradrenaline is concentrated in chromaffin granules in the nerve terminals by an uptake process which is Na^+-dependent. The level of free noradrenaline in the cytoplasm is controlled by the mitochondrial enzyme monoamine oxidase (MAO) of which there are several types with differing substrate affinities. Action potentials arriving in the terminals cause an influx of Ca^{2+} which evokes the release of noradrenaline by a process of exocytosis. Released noradrenaline may interact with postsynaptic receptors and some is removed in the circulation, ultimately to be methy-lated by catechol-0-methyl transferase and deaminated by MAO. However, most of the released noradrenaline is avidly taken up again by the terminals by a high-affinity, saturable, re-uptake process called uptake 1. In addition some is taken up by another low-affinity uptake system, called uptake 2, located postsynap-tically. Most of the amine taken up by the terminals by uptake 1

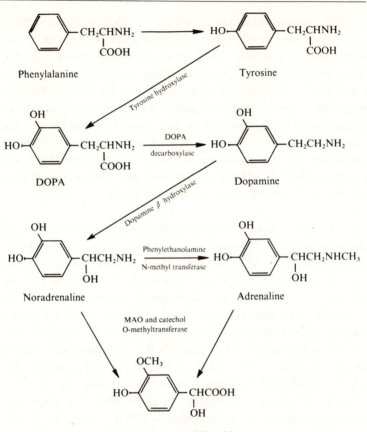

3-methoxy-4-hydroxy mandelic acid

Fig. 3.4. Metabolic pathways for catecholamines.

is re-incorporated into the granules, although some is inactivated by MAO. Thus the system may operate economically at a relatively low rate of de-novo synthesis of noradrenaline.

Many therapeutically useful drugs and many of research interest interfere in a relatively selective fashion with one or more of these processes.

Tyramine is a sympathomimetic drug which exerts its effects indirectly by precipitating the release of the endogenous transmitter noradrenaline. It is a substrate for uptake 1 across the terminal membrane and enters the granules to displace noradrenaline from its storage site in sufficient quantity to cause postsynaptic actions. Since tyramine is a substrate for MAO it is likely that it acts as a substrate competitor with noradrenaline, so enabling noradrenaline released into the cytoplasm to be released before it is inactivated by MAO. MAO converts tyramine into octopamine which may be stored in the granules and neurally released as a 'false transmitter'.

Tyramine is present in many foodstuffs in considerable quantities, e.g. some cheeses, but after ingestion is largely destroyed by MAO in the liver and intestines. However, in patients treated with MAO inhibitors this protective mechanism is inactivated and the taking of foodstuffs containing large quantities of tyramine may precipitate a crisis due to the resulting high blood pressure and consequent cerebral oedema and haemorrhage. The peripheral sympathomimetic effects of the central stimulant *amphetamine* are produced in a similar fashion.

The peripheral effects of indirectly acting sympathomimetics are prevented by pretreatment with *reserpine* which causes a rapid and prolonged depletion of noradrenaline stores by blocking the pumping mechanism of the granule membrane. It does not affect uptake 1. Reserpine causes a depletion of noradrenaline and 5-hydroxytryptamine at the periphery and in the CNS. It has been widely used as a tranquilliser and as a hypotensive agent but its usefulness is limited by the fact that it causes severe depression, sometimes with suicidal tendencies and other drugs which lack these effects are clearly to be preferred.

Guanethidine, a widely used and potent antihypertensive drug, causes a slow depletion of noradrenaline from the granule store and is concentrated by the terminals. However, the hypotensive action occurs before any detectable change in the levels of noradrenaline in the terminals. Furthermore, there is not a good correlation between hypotensive effect and depletion of noradrenaline in a series of drugs chemically related to guanethidine. It is probable that the early hypotensive effects of guanethidine are due to a blockade of the neural release mechanism, and that the depletion of transmitter may serve to prolong the effect. The slow depletion of noradrenaline may be due to a neurotoxic effect causing a degeneration of nerve terminals.

Bretylium was introduced as an antihypertensive agent shortly before guanethidine but it rapidly produces tolerance which limits its usefulness, Bretylium does not cause a depletion of the noradrenaline stores but more directly prevents the release of transmitter.

α-methyldopa is converted to α-methyl noradrenaline which is stored and may be released as a 'false-transmitter' by neural stimulation. It was at first considered that this was the mechanism of its antihypertensive effect. This seems unlikely because α-methyl noradrenaline is not greatly different in potency from noradrenaline itself. A more probable explanation is that α-methyl DOPA exerts its therapeutic effects by an action on the central nervous system.

Uptake 1 is selectively blocked by the antidepressant compounds *imipramine* and amitriptyline. It is also blocked by cocaine but not by other local anaesthetics. A block of uptake 1 leads to a potentiation of the effects of systemically administered noradrenaline. Adrenaline is not as good a substrate for uptake 1 as is noradrenaline and is potentiated to a lesser degree, while isoprenaline is a very poor substrate and is unaffected.

The recent emphasis on presynaptic receptors for acetylcholine and catecholamines on noradrenergic terminals suggests that many more drugs may influence the release of catecholamines.

Peripheral cholinergic synapses

All postganglionic parasympathetic nerves cholinergically innervate their effector organs. The chief outflows from the CNS are in cranial nerves III, VII, IX and X and in the sacral pelvic nerves. The occulomotor nerve (III) causes constriction of the pupil. Cranial nerves VII and IX supply the lachrimal and salivary glands to evoke secretions. The vagus nerves innervate most of the viscera including heart, lungs, trachea and bronchi, liver, spleen, stomach, intestines and kidneys and cause effects ranging from increases in motility of the gastrointestinal tract to slowing of the heart. There are also a few postganglionic cholinergic sympathetic fibres which cause vasodilatation of some blood vessels and innervate the sweat glands. The sacral pelvic nerves innervate the urinary bladder and its internal sphincter and the rectum.

At all of these sites the ACh receptors appear to be of the muscarinic type and are therefore activated by muscarine, acetyl-β-methylcholine, pilocarpine and arecoline. Antagonists are atropine, methyl-atropine, dibutoline and lachesine. These agents are all reversible competitive antagonists of ACh at muscarinic receptors. Benzilylcholine mustard combines non-reversibly with the receptor and for this reason has been extremely useful in identifying muscarinic receptors.

Botulinum toxin prevents the release of ACh from autonomic cholinergic terminals, just as it does at motor nerve terminals, and so causes a paralysis of the parasympathetic nervous system.

Although atropine effectively prevents the action of exo-genously administered ACh on tissues which have a cholinergic innervation from the autonomic nervous system, it is not always effective in completely blocking the effects of electrical stimulation of parasympathetic nerves. One, now classic, example of such an atropine-resistant effect is the early contraction of the urinary bladder evoked by stimulation of the pelvic nerves. In contrast, the vagal effects on the heart are completely counteracted by atropine. The explanation of such atropine-resistant actions is not completely certain. It may be that ACh is at first released in such large quantities or in such close proximity to the receptors that the concentration of atropine administered is inadequate to compete effectively at the receptors. An unlikely possibility is that there are perisynaptic barriers which prevent the access of atropine. It is also possible that ACh is not the only substance liberated and it has been suggested that some nerves are purinergic in function.

Anticholinesterase drugs reproduce the effects of ACh on muscarinic receptors. They cause constriction of the pupil and a decrease in intra-ocular pressure, a property which has found some application in the treatment of glaucoma. They increase gastrointestinal motility and this action may be useful in the treatment of atonic conditions of the bowel and urinary bladder. Anticholinesterase drugs also cause copious secretions from the salivary and lachrimal glands.

Thus, in general the pharmacology of postganglionic cholinergic transmission is relatively straightforward and will not be covered in any more detail in this account. The interested reader is referred to the relevant chapters in Goodman and Gilman (1975) for a detailed discussion of parasympathetic substances and their antagonists.

CHAPTER FOUR

Techniques used to study transmitters and drug action in the CNS

The investigation of drug action in the CNS is beset by a number of problems including how to get the drug to its site of action in the brain, how to monitor the activity of the drug and how to interpret the pharmacological actions observed in terms of the clinical effects of the drug.

Since many of the drugs influence neurotransmitter mechanisms it is necessary to know the nature of the transmitters and their relationship to anatomical structures and pathways, and techniques are being continuously refined in order to answer these questions.

ROUTES OF DRUG ADMINISTRATION

Systemic administration

The easiest way in which to administer a drug is into the general circulation. Intravenous injection has the advantage that it is not only easy to perform but that the blood levels can be ascertained and a comparison made between concentrations necessary to produce a given pharmacological action and concentrations which are effective in man. The drug must of course pass through the blood–brain barrier but this would not be a serious objection in the study of clinically useful drugs because they must in any case cross the barrier to produce therapeutic effects on the CNS. However, in the study of CNS transmitters, which do not generally cross the blood–brain barrier with ease, intravenous injection is of less value.

There are serious disadvantages with systemic administration when attempting to define the locus and mechanism of drug effects with any precision, because the drug may be exerting its effect indirectly on that part of the CNS being studied: it may even be producing an effect on the CNS by modifying peripheral function and thus changing the inflow of sensory information.

The time course of drug action after intravenous injection may be relatively prolonged. Although this may not be a serious disadvantage in some situations, e.g. in the study of drug effects on animal behaviour, in electrophysiological studies with micro-electrodes, the period for which stable recordings can be obtained may often be rather limited and systemic administration may severely limit the amount of data which can be obtained.

Local administration

A more restricted locus of drug action can be achieved by a variety of techniques. These include injection into the cerebro-spinal fluid (CSF), local perfusion of superficial parts of the brain or local perfusion of deeper areas by a 'push–pull' technique, microinjection or microelectrophoresis. Of these various methods, microelectrophoresis attains the most restricted site of drug action because the drugs are administered from a micro-pipette in close vicinity to the site at which electrical recordings are being obtained. In order to do this, ionised drugs are ejected from the micropipettes by the passage of a small electric current usually within the range of $0–100 \times 10^{-9}$ A, through the solution. Even this widely used technique has disadvantages in that the precise concentration at the site of action is not known, even though the amount being administered in unit time can be ascertained. Furthermore, as with all techniques utilising local administration, the concentration of drug achieved will be highest at the site of application and will decrease rapidly with distance. In one sense, this is an advantage but if the administration of the drug is severely restricted to a very small part of a neurone then effects at distant synapses on that same neurone may be difficult to detect.

In general, it may be concluded that no one technique is ideal but that the most useful and conclusive data will be obtained when several techniques have been employed producing consistent results.

Further refinements in techniques of recording from isolated sections of nervous tissue are currently under way and should enable the effects of known concentrations of drugs to be studied on relatively small parts of the brain. It is to be anticipated that although this relatively new technique may well give new insight into the mode of action of drugs and transmitters upon neuronal membranes, the unphysiological nature of the preparation and in particular its separation from functionally related areas of the nervous system will limit its usefulness.

BEHAVIOURAL TECHNIQUES

Behavioural techniques have been widely employed, particularly in the early evaluation of potentially useful new drugs. Although it may be possible to interpret such experiments in psychological terms, it is certainly difficult to interpret them in precise terms of locus and mechanism of action because the interrelationship between psychological parameters of behaviour and detailed physiology and anatomy is rather imprecise. A detailed consideration of this complex subject is beyond the scope of this book and the interested reader is referred to the book on *Behavioural Pharmacology* by Iversen and Iversen (1975).

BIOCHEMICAL AND HISTOCHEMICAL TECHNIQUES

A great deal of our knowledge of the location and distribution of central synaptic transmitters and their associated enzymes can be attributed to the work of biochemists and histologists. Some of the more important aspects of this subject are covered in the chapter on central neurotransmitters and only a summary of the available techniques is presented here.

At the first level of investigation it has been shown that different neurotransmitters are present in different concentrations in different regions of the brain. In general, those areas which contain the highest concentration of a particular neurotransmitter also contain the highest concentrations of synthesising enzymes. However, the distribution of the degradative enzymes does not necessarily correlate well with these distributions, possibly because these enzymes may not always be specifically involved in the inactivation of that transmitter.

Drug effects on the levels of transmitters in various regions of the brain have been frequently reported. In general, these are difficult to interpret because it is often not known what is cause and what is effect of a change in function. Nevertheless, such studies, coupled with studies on turnover of the transmitter, its release or the production of metabolites may provide the first clues to the mechanism of drug effects, particularly when restricted to just one neurotransmitter system.

At the present time there is great emphasis on data obtained on binding studies of drugs and neurotransmitters to isolated brain components and such studies are providing important new information on drug action, even though they are also frequently difficult to extrapolate to the whole animal and in particular to therapeutic effects.

Some of the most elegant demonstrations of the location of neurotransmitters and the neurones which utilise them have been made with histochemical and immunohistochemical techniques. Such studies have provided great impetus to the electrophysiologists and 'micropharmacologists' in providing indications of just where to administer drugs and make recordings.

ELECTROPHYSIOLOGICAL TECHNIQUES

The electrical activity of the nervous system can be observed in many ways. It is a relatively simple matter to record a spinal reflex from a peripheral motor nerve and to show changes after the administration of drugs. Such observations have rather limited value because they tell us little about how a drug causes that effect. The recording of the electrical activity of large areas of the brain, expressed either as electroencephalograms (EEG's) or evoked potentials has also been greatly employed and may be of some value in diagnosis of disorders or in predicting possible clinical applications of new drugs. However, EEG's and evoked potentials can tell us little about precise localisation or mechanism of drug effects.

Electrophysiological studies with microelectrode recordings from single neurones of known synaptic connections and functions, coupled with the microelectrophoretic administration of drugs to such neurones has probably been of greatest value in assessing the mechanism of action of neurotransmitters, particularly when intracellular recording techniques have been employed. These techniques have also been of value in helping to identify the nature of the neurotransmitter at some synapses but they have not been a striking success in demonstrating how many important therapeutic agents achieve their results, although they have been instrumental in defining the action of some toxic substances such as strychnine, tetanus toxin and nicotine.

CONCLUSIONS

It must therefore be concluded that no one technique is likely to provide definitive answers to the problems of drug action on the central nervous system. The multifaceted approach, combining studies in the various disciplines, each with their own limitations, has nevertheless provided a plethora of facts which in some instances has gelled into a reasonably satisfying hypothesis of the mechanisms of drug action. At other times, the limitations of the techniques have provided data which are difficult to reconcile and it is these which provide the greatest challenge to the enquiring mind.

CHAPTER FIVE

Central neurotransmitters

INTRODUCTION

Of the many drugs which act upon the central nervous system, most appear to do so by an effect upon synaptic transmission. In the evolution of the nervous system it seems that a variety of chemical substances have assumed the role of chemical mediator and to a variable extent some of these have become associated with particular functions, although there is considerable overlap. Perhaps as a consequence of this specialisation, derangement of neuronal functions may sometimes be associated with defects in the operation of one transmitter system whilst others appear to operate in a more or less normal fashion. Drugs which act in the most selective fashion are therefore likely to be those with the most specific site of action on a process which in turn is relatively specific for a particular transmitter. Such drugs could act either by modifying selective binding of the transmitter to its receptor site or by effects on the synthesis, degradation or release of the transmitter. The overlapping functions of neuronal pathways utilising the same transmitter leads to the generalisation that drugs selectively operating upon a transmitter system may affect a number of functions not all of which are necessarily deranged in disease.

The topography of the connections of neurones employing different transmitters, a knowledge of changes which occur in disease states and an understanding of the mechanism of action of useful drugs may therefore lead to a rational approach to therapy.

Over the last few decades there have been many advances in the development and application of techniques for the identification of central neurotransmitters and for mapping their presence in the CNS, coupled with advances in neurophysiological and micropharmacological methods which have led to a greater

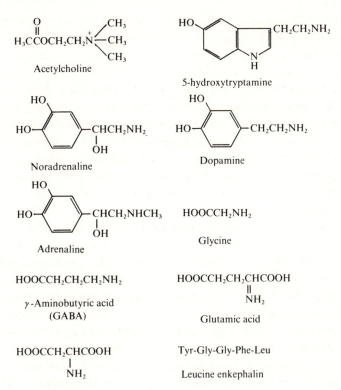

Fig. 5.1. Central neurotransmitters.

understanding of central neurotransmitters. Fig. 5.1 lists a number of endogenous substances which are currently under consideration as neurotransmitters in the CNS.

In order to establish the identity of a neurotransmitter it is necessary to fully substantiate only two criteria. The first is that the putative transmitter is released when the presynaptic nerve is stimulated and the second is that the putative transmitter, when administered as an exogenous substance to the postsynaptic neurone, reproduces exactly the effect of the endogenously released substance. Close examination of this statement reveals that it embodies a number of accessory assumptions which will provide a partial solution to the question, 'is substance X a transmitter?' If a substance can be released then it must be assumed to be present and probably synthesised. Thus much of the supporting evidence for the identity of a particular transmitter is based upon demonstrations of the presence and distribution of the substance and its associated synthetic or degradative enzymes within the CNS. Release of the substance when particular pathways within the brain are activated is technically more difficult to demonstrate, but this has been done in many instances.

Identity of action of exogenously administered and endogenously released neurotransmitter embodies a number of subsidiary considerations, all of which are capable of experimental verification. There are two which are probably most informative. The first is the demonstration that the pharmacology of the exogenous substance is identical to that of the endogenous transmitter. Pharmacological observations within this category are likely to include structure–activity studies with agonists, studies with specific receptor antagonists, enzyme activators or inactivators, uptake inhibitors etc. The second is that the precise membrane mechanism by which the transmitter causes excitation or inhibition is identified in both instances. Almost inevitably, most investigations of this type will be electrophysiological in nature. Such evidence is most complete for the inhibitory transmitter glycine. Subsidiary evidence relating to the mechanisms of action can be derived from binding studies and such biochemical studies as enzyme activation, as in the example of dopamine-activated adenylate cyclase, or inactivation.

ACETYLCHOLINE

Acetylcholine is found in many parts of the brain, especially high concentrations being found in the caudate nucleus and cerebral cortex. In general, the distribution of the transmitter corresponds to the distribution of choline acetyltransferase and of the muscarinic cholinergic receptor.

In order to study the topography of cholinergic neurones a sensitive technique for visualising either acetylcholine or choline acetyltransferase is urgently required but so far has not been developed. The most promising approach at present being developed is an immunohistochemical technique for the enzyme but some increase in specificity is necessary.

A histochemical technique for visualising nerve tracts containing acetylcholinesterase has been developed and extensive maps obtained. However, there are a number of esterases and they may not all function in neurotransmission and such maps cannot be interpreted without supporting evidence. In particular, acetylcholinesterase occurs in a high concentration in cerebellum, and nerve fibres containing the enzyme have been demonstrated with the copper-thiocholine technique. However, there is little acetylcholine, choline acetyltransferase or cholinergic receptor material in cerebellum and neurophysiological evidence of cholinergic transmission is lacking.

Acetylcholine usually excites central neurones when administered by microelectrophoresis, but inhibitory effects have also been shown, especially in nucleus reticularis of the thalamus and in the brain stem. There is some neurophysiological evidence for cholinergic pathways to the cerebral cortex and hippocampus but in general precise definition of the pathways is not yet possible.

The synapse formed by the termination of collaterals of motor axons on Renshaw cells in the spinal cord is the best characterised site of cholinergic transmission in the CNS (Fig. 5.2). Here, the action of acetylcholine released from presynaptic terminals of the axon collaterals exerts a short latency monosynaptic excitatory action on the Renshaw cell followed by a long-latency, prolonged period of excitation with a different mechanism. The short-latency excitation causes cell firing lasting for about 50 ms and is blocked by pharmacological agents which block nicotinic receptors for acetylcholine, such as dihydro-β-erythroidine and d-tubocurarine, and is prolonged by inhibitors of cholinesterase.

The major action of acetylcholine administered microelectrophoretically is also due to excitation of nicotinic receptors. The release of acetylcholine is blocked by the administration of botulinus toxin and direct assays from perfusates of spinal cords

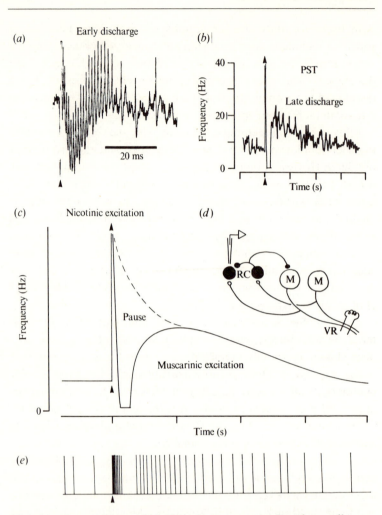

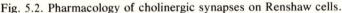

Fig. 5.2. Pharmacology of cholinergic synapses on Renshaw cells.

Stimulation (arrows) of the ventral root (VR) with single electric shocks gives rise to excitatory–inhibitory–excitatory sequences in Renshaw cells (RC). The motoneurones (M) have axons which branch within the grey matter to form collaterals which synapse on Renshaw cells. ACh is liberated to interact first with nicotinic receptors, the activation of which evokes repetitive action potentials (early discharge) lasting for about 50 ms (a). The action potentials occur at about 1 ms intervals (frequency 1 KHz) at the beginning of the discharge. The early discharge is attenuated by dihydro-β-erythroidine which competitively antagonises the effect of ACh on nicotinic receptors.

The full sequence of events is shown schematically in (e) and as a have demonstrated an increased release after antidromic stimulation of ventral roots. The nicotinic actions of acetylcholine released by stimulation of motor axons or applied from micropipettes is potentiated by the administration of inhibitors of acetylcholinesterase. The long-latency excitation after antidromic stimulation of ventral roots lasts for up to 5 s and is due to the interaction of released acetylcholine with muscarinic receptors because it is antagonised by atropine, well-known for its ability to block peripheral muscarinic receptors. After blockade of nicotinic receptors with dihydro-β-erythroidine a muscarinic action can be demonstrated by the iontophoresis of acetyl-β-methylcholine or muscarine.

The membrane mechanisms of the action of acetylcholine on Renshaw cells have not been clearly elucidated although nicotinic effects appear to be associated with an increase in membrane conductance.

Muscarinic actions of acetylcholine are the most prominent elsewhere in the nervous system. Krnjevic has shown that the muscarinic excitatory effect on cerebral cortical neurones is associated with a depolarisation and a decreased membrane conductance, probably reflecting a selective decrease in permeability to potassium ions.

AMINO ACIDS

There are three amino acids commonly considered to be transmitters in the CNS. These are glycine, gamma-amino-butyric acid (GABA) and glutamic acid. Selective antagonists are available for

peristimulus histogram on the same time scale in (c). The record in (b) is from an actual experiment. The histograms are computed from several repetitions of the stimulus on the same cell and represent the average firing frequency at various times before and after the stimulus.

The early discharge is followed by a 'pause', during which the excitatory background activity is suppressed. The pause is due to a combination of mutual inhibitory connections between the Renshaw cells, where the transmitter is probably glycine, and to desensitisation. The late discharge follows the pause and has a prolonged time course lasting for several seconds. It is not blocked by dihydro-β-erythroidine but is abolished by atropine, a competitive antagonist of ACh at muscarinic sites.

glycine and GABA and the evidence that these are transmitters at certain sites is strong. Antagonists for glutamic acid have been found, but they are probably insufficiently selective for the evidence derived from studies with them to be as convincing as would be desirable. Nevertheless, there remains good evidence that glutamic acid is a transmitter. Some other amino acids, such as taurine and aspartic acid, have also occasionally been proposed as transmitters but the evidence for this is weak.

Glutamic acid is ubiquitous in the central nervous system and serves metabolic as well as transmitter functions. When applied by microelectrophoresis to nerve cells it causes a depolarisation, due to an increased permeability to sodium ions. Depolarisation is usually sufficient to increase the firing rate of neurones.

Glycine is distributed mainly in the spinal cord and medullary parts of the brain stem. It invariably inhibits neurones by increasing membrane permeability to chloride and potassium ions, causing a hyperpolarisation. It is the mediator of postsynaptic inhibition at a number of identified synapses, including the recurrent inhibitory synapses of Renshaw cells upon motoneurones, the inhibitory synapses of interneurones mediating reciprocal IA inhibition on motoneurones and on Renshaw cells and the inhibitory synapses on motoneurones of interneurones excited by IB fibres from Golgi tendon organs. Strychnine and some related drugs are specific receptor antagonists and has been shown to interact with glycine at binding sites in in-vitro systems. The inhibitory effect of glycine is generally more marked on spinal neurones than on supraspinal neurones and it probably acts as a postsynaptic inhibitory transmitter mainly at spinal cord synapses.

In contrast, GABA and its associated enzymes are found in higher concentrations in supraspinal than in spinal regions of the CNS. At supraspinal sites it has been identified as the postsynaptic inhibitory transmitter, acting by a membrane mechanism indistinguishable from that of glycine, at a number of synapses. In the spinal cord it is the most likely mediator of presynaptic inhibition in which afferent terminals become depolarised and transmission reduced by a mechanism which is the subject of considerable controversy. Antagonists of the inhibitory actions of GABA on spinal and supraspinal neurones and of presynaptic inhibition are picrotoxin and bicuculline.

Visualisation of GABA-containing neurones has been more successful than visualisation of glutamate or glycine containing neurones. Autoradiography, in which labelled amino acid is taken up by a tissue followed by photographic determination of the distribution in a tissue slice, has been extensively used but suffers from the disadvantage that the amino acids may be taken up not only by neurones but also by glial cells. More recently, a sensitive immunohistochemical method for glutamic acid decarboxylase (GAD), which forms GABA from its precursor glutamic acid, has been successfully used to confirm the presence of specific 'GABA-utilising' pathways in the CNS.

CATECHOLAMINES AND 5-HYDROXYTRYPTAMINE

The first highly successful demonstrations of pathways in the CNS containing noradrenaline (NA), dopamine (DA) and 5-hydroxytryptamine (5-HT) were made with a fluorescence technique in which tissue sections are treated with formaldehyde vapour under carefully controlled conditions to form fluorescent isoquinolines. Later investigations with an immunohistochemical technique for dopamine-β-hydroxylase have confirmed the original observations for NA made with the fluorescence method. In more recent studies condensation with glyoxylic acid is used to form fluorescent products.

Major dopaminergic pathways (the nigrostriatal and mesolimbic systems) originate from the region of the substantia nigra and ventral tegmental area and project principally to the basal ganglia, limbic system and cerebral cortex (Fig. 5.3). Another pathway (the tuberoinfundibular system) originates from cells of the arcuate nucleus and projects mainly to the median eminence of the hypothalamus.

Noradrenergic pathways are more diffuse with cell bodies in the pons and medulla, including a localised group of neurones in the locus coeruleus. There are rostral projections to many parts of the brain and caudal projections to the spinal cord.

Microelectrophoretic administration of NA to CNS neurones

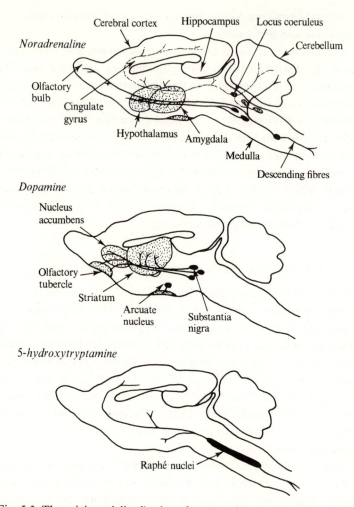

Fig. 5.3. The origin and distribution of monoaminergic fibres in the brain. Noradrenaline and dopamine pathways redrawn after Livett, B. G. (1973) *Brit. Med. Bull.*, **29**, 93.

usually causes inhibition but excitatory effects have also been demonstrated. There have been rather few studies of the membrane mechanism affected by NA but there is some indication that the inhibitory effect is associated with a hyperpolarisation and an increase in membrane resistance. There is also some evidence that, at least in cerebellum, the effect may be mediated via cyclic AMP.

It might be expected that agents which antagonise the effects of NA at peripheral α- and β-receptors might also act in the CNS. Although antagonism has been demonstrated in some studies, it has not been possible to demonstrate specific effects in others.

This relative lack of potent, reliable and specific antagonists at central sites has hindered the conclusive demonstration of noradrenergic transmission at identified central synapses.

Although the amount of adrenaline in the CNS is small relative to that of NA, the presence of phenylethanolamine-N-methyltransferase has been demonstrated and specific immunohistochemical methods have led to preliminary indications of adrenergic transmission with a rather restricted distribution.

5-HT is located in the cell bodies of neurones predominantly situated in the raphé nuclei in the brain stem. The tryptaminergic neurones project both rostrally and caudally into the spinal cord. Although an immunohistochemical technique is available for DOPA-decarboxylase, the enzyme responsible for the decarboxylation of DOPA is immunologically indistinguishable from that which decarboxylates 5-hydroxytryptophan and so is of limited usefulness.

5-HT may either excite or inhibit neurones when it is administered microelectrophoretically. Lysergic acid diethylamide and related substances have been found to antagonise these effects in some investigations but not in others. It has been suggested that 5-HT systems may be important as a 'trigger' system for slow-wave sleep whereas noradrenergic systems originating from the locus coeruleus are involved in 'deep' or 'paradoxical' sleep.

POLYPEPTIDES

It has long been known that the polypeptide, substance P occurs in the CNS and is localised in the synaptosomal fractions of brain homogenates with a subcellular distribution similar to that of acetylcholine. More recently, immunological techniques have been employed to demonstrate the presence of particularly high concentrations especially in the dorsal grey matter of the spinal cord and in the caudate nucleus.

Another group of polypeptides, namely the enkephalins, have also been shown to have rather specific distributions. There is also evidence for nerve terminals containing other polypeptides such as neurotoxin, somatostatin and thyrotrophin releasing factor (TRF) in the central nervous system.

Microelectrophoretic studies with synthetic polypeptides have shown that they are potent excitants or depressants of neurones in the CNS but further elucidation of their function at specific synapses awaits future developments.

CHAPTER SIX

General anaesthetics

INTRODUCTION

The general anaesthetics comprise a large group of compounds of diverse chemical structure which cause a loss of sensation and perception leading in adequate doses to a complete, but reversible loss of consciousness. Although they may cause an attenuation of pain sensation in subanaesthetic doses, this is not invariably so, and the anaesthetics as a class are distinct from the analgesic drugs which selectively reduce the sensation of pain but do not lead to a loss of consciousness at therapeutic concentrations.

The general anaesthetics depress function at all levels of the central nervous system and so may depress respiration, circulation, temperature control, voluntary reflex movements and pain, but the degree of depression of each of these functions is not the same with all agents, even at a similar depth of anaesthesia. It therefore follows that the characteristics of anaesthesia with different agents may vary.

TYPES OF GENERAL ANAESTHETIC

The chemical structures of a variety of different general anaesthetics are given in Fig. 6.1. The diversity of structures is readily apparent and must be taken into consideration in evaluating the mechanisms of action. The physical form of anaesthetics also varies from gaseous substances such as the inert gases, nitrous oxide and cyclopropane, or volatile substances such as ether, chloroform and halothane, to soluble substances typified by the barbiturates, eugenols, steroid anaesthetics and cyclohexylamine. To a large degree, the physical form and properties of the anaesthetic determine the manner in which the anaesthetic is used, and some of the advantages and disadvantages of each class.

Gaseous :	Nitrous oxide	N_2O
	Cyclopropane	

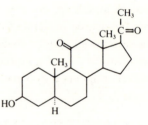

Volatile :	Diethyl ether	$CH_3CH_2OCH_2CH_3$
	Chloroform	$CHCl_3$
	Halothane	$CF_3CHClBr$
	Methoxyfluorane	$CH_3OCF_2CHCl_2$

Soluble (intravenous) :

	Barbiturates (fig. 6.2)	

O—CH₂CON (C₂H₅)₂

Propanidid (a eugenol)

$CH_2COOCH_2CH_2CH_3$

Alphaxalone

Ketamine

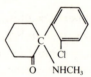

Fig. 6.1. General anaesthetics.

Gaseous anaesthetics

Nitrous oxide was the first anaesthetic to be used in clinical practice in the middle of the nineteenth century, although its use was closely followed by that of the volatile anaesthetics, chloroform and ether.

At atmospheric pressure, nitrous oxide has a rather low

anaesthetic potency. It is administered by inhalation and to achieve adequate depths of anaesthesia the concentration in inspired air must be increased to such a level that anoxia and cyanosis ensues. Used alone, for example in dentistry, it can therefore only be administered for very brief periods. However, at subanaesthetic concentrations it has good analgesic properties and so is often used to supplement anaesthesia induced by other agents. At the higher atmospheric pressures which can be achieved in hyperbaric chambers, nitrous oxide may be used to achieve anaesthesia at concentrations mixed with oxygen which do not cause anoxia.

Cyclopropane is another gaseous anaesthetic administered by inhalation. It has a higher anaesthetic potency than nitrous oxide and so does not cause anoxia. However, it is an explosive gas and its use has declined in more recent years.

Both nitrous oxide and cyclopropane have a low solubility in blood such that a rapid equilibrium is achieved between the concentration in the inspired gas mixture and the blood. Consequently the concentration in the alveolus is not greatly reduced during each inspiration and the rate of equilibration of blood and lung concentrations is chiefly determined by the cardiac output, rather than the rate and depth of respiration. The induction of anaesthesia is therefore rapid because the rate of equilibration between blood and brain is not a limiting factor.

Volatile anaesthetics

Ether, chloroform, halothane and related drugs may be vaporised at room temperature by passing a stream of gas over the surface of the liquid. The degree of vaporisation and the concentration in the administered gas mixture is determined mainly by the temperature, and adequate means of controlling temperature or compensating for changes are necessary if reproducible concentrations in the gas mixture are to be obtained.

The volatile anaesthetics are all more soluble in blood than nitrous oxide or cyclopropane. The solubility is such that during each inspiration the concentration of gas in the alveoli is greatly diminished.

The rate of attainment of equilibrium between blood concentration, and therefore tension in blood, and the concentration in the inspired gas mixture is therefore slow and determined by the rate and depth of respiration, rather than by the cardiac output. It has been estimated that 90% equilibration of the blood with diethylether administered at a constant concentration requires about 20 h of administration. The equivalent time for nitrous oxide would be about 1 h. If highly soluble volatile anaesthetics were to be administered at concentrations just sufficient for anaesthesia at equilibrium then the induction of anaesthesia would be an extremely slow process. This disadvantage can be overcome by one of two methods. First, the concentration of inspired gas during the first stages of induction is greatly in excess of that which would cause anaesthesia at equilibrium. An anaesthetic concentration in blood is therefore rapidly attained. The concentration in the inspired air may then be gradually reduced towards the equilibrium concentration as anaesthesia progresses. The rate of onset of anaesthesia may also be accelerated by increasing the rate of respiration, e.g. by the administration of increased concentrations of carbon dioxide in the gas mixture.

The plateau principle states that at equilibrium the rate of administration of a substance is equal to the rate of elimination. It therefore follows that anaesthetics which only slowly attain equilibrium concentrations in blood will also be eliminated at a slow rate. This is clearly a major disadvantage with anaesthetics from which rapid and complete recovery is usually desirable to avoid post-operative complications. In addition such drugs are highly lipid soluble. During prolonged periods of administration they will therefore be accumulated by body fat. The rate of attainment of equilibrium between blood and fat is a slow process due to the fact that blood flow in the body fat is a rate limiting process. There will therefore be a rather prolonged 'hangover' effect if the duration of administration is sufficiently prolonged to cause significant increases in the concentration of anaesthetic in the body fat, from which it will be even more slowly eliminated, with consequent maintained low levels of anaesthetic in the blood.

Ether is an inflammable, and therefore dangerous, anaesthetic. It is very irritant to the respiratory mucosa and causes copious secretions and may cause laryngospasm. It causes less respiratory depression than chloroform and may cause intense excitement during the early stages of induction. Its major advantage is that it is an inexpensive anaesthetic.

Chloroform is not inflammable but is particularly liable to cause liver damage.

Halothane is a relatively modern drug which was synthesised in a deliberate effort to achieve a non-inflammable and safe volatile anaesthetic. It is less prone to cause liver damage than chloroform in normal use but repeated exposure, as may be experienced by the anaesthetist, may have toxic effects on the liver. It has analgesic properties and produces a smooth induction of anaesthesia with minimal excitement. However, it causes a marked circulatory depression at anaesthetic concentrations. It also causes some respiratory depression. Circulatory depression is less marked with the related anaesthetic, methoxyfluorane, but respiratory depression is more evident with this agent.

Many anaesthetics, including cyclopropane, chloroform, halothane and methoxyfluorane appear to sensitise the myocardium to circulating catecholamines and may cause ventricular fibrillation.

Soluble (intravenous) anaesthetics

Von Bayer synthesised barbituric acid by condensing together urea and malonic acid in 1864. Barbituric acid is not itself an anaesthetic but is the parent of a long line of derivatives which are. The first of these was sodium barbitone, synthesised by Fischer and Von Mering in 1903, but its action is too prolonged for modern use. Phenobarbitone was synthesised in 1912. It is also quite long-acting and used more as a sedative and anti-epileptic in subanaesthetic doses, rather than as an anaesthetic.

The first really useful, short-acting barbiturate was thiopentone, introduced during the Second World War. The introduction of this substance led to relatively safe and short-lasting anaesthesia.

The structures of some of the more important barbiturates are shown in Fig. 6.2. In clinical anaesthesia only those with the shortest duration of action, e.g. thiopentone, methohexitone and thiohexitone are widely used.

The duration of the anaesthetic effect is governed by two

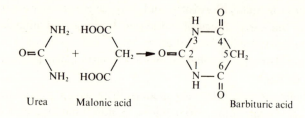

Urea   Malonic acid   Barbituric acid

Anaesthetics derived from barbituric acid by substitution in
positions 2, 3, 5 :

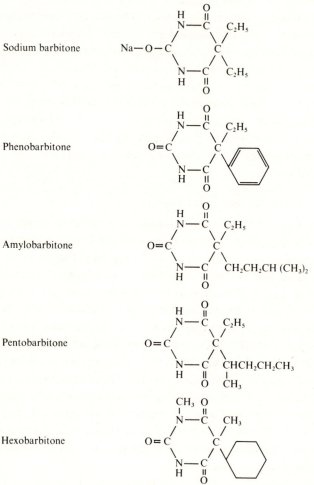

Sodium barbitone

Phenobarbitone

Amylobarbitone

Pentobarbitone

Hexobarbitone

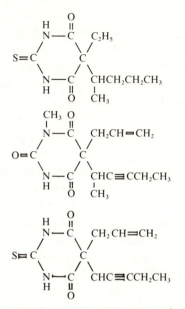

Thiopentone

Methohexitone

Thiohexitone

Fig. 6.2. Barbiturates. (Anaesthetics are listed in order of decreasing duration of effect.)

factors which determine the plasma level. Redistribution of the drug is probably the most important factor with thiopentone, whereas metabolism becomes rate limiting for methohexitone and thiohexitone, although redistribution still occurs. Redistribution in body tissues which are well perfused by blood, e.g. muscle, are more important than redistribution into body fat, which is poorly perfused by blood, even though the drugs have a high fat:plasma partition coefficient.

The high fat solubility of the barbiturates leads to a good absorption from the gastrointestinal tract. However, they are not administered by this route for anaesthesia because the ratio between toxic and therapeutic plasma concentrations is too small and absorption too unreliable for this route of administration to be safe. Nevertheless, when used as sedatives or hypnotics in subanaesthetic concentrations, the oral route is relatively safe and certainly more convenient than intravenous injection.

Eugenols such as propanidid are esters and rapidly hydrolysed by plasma and liver esterases. They are therefore extremely short-acting and have been used for out-patients. Unlike the barbiturates, they rarely cause laryngospasm or bronchospasm.

The soluble steroidal anaesthetics such as alphaxalone are also short-acting anaesthetics which cause good muscle relaxation.

Cyclohexylamine ('Ketamine') produces a rather unusual type of anaesthesia, sometimes called 'dissociative' anaesthesia. The drug was developed from a series of psychotomimetic substances and the use of the first of these with anaesthetic properties, phencyclidine, had to be abandoned because of the severity and prolonged nature of its psychological side-effects which included hallucinations and mania lasting for days. These effects are less marked and prolonged with ketamine but during induction the patient may experience odd sensations or even frank hallucinations. The muscles are not relaxed during anaesthesia, and the limbs may move involuntarily, but reflexes to painful stimuli are attenuated. The major advantage of ketamine is that it causes minimal effects on the cardiovascular system and may therefore be particularly indicated in those patients with cardiac disease or in the elderly.

In general, the short-acting intravenous anaesthetics are used for induction of anaesthesia because they cause a smooth and rapid induction, with minimal stress or excitement. However, the anaesthesia is usually maintained during more prolonged surgery by the administration of a volatile or gaseous anaesthetic, or combinations of these, often with additional analgesic drugs and other agents.

MECHANISMS OF ANAESTHESIA

Physico-chemical theories

The great diversity in the chemical structures of substances causing anaesthesia, ranging from the inert gases to such complex molecules as steroids, renders it improbable that anaesthesia is explicable in terms of interaction with a single, specific receptor molecule. In this respect the anaesthetics comprise a class of compounds differing from all of the others discussed in this book.

A certain natural tendency to search for a single explanation for the phenomenon of anaesthesia has led to several physico-chemical theories of anaesthetic action based upon some non-specific action of the substances upon cell membranes.

While such theories have the merit of simplicity and rather precise supporting data, they often fail to account for certain discrepancies in the data and pay no heed to the qualitatively different aspects of anaesthesia with different agents. Purely physico-chemical effects upon cell membranes may indeed be an adequate explanation of some of the chemically simpler anaesthetics, but the apparent correlations between anaesthetic potency and physico-chemical parameters for more complex molecules may simply reflect the physical environment in which the anaesthetic acts, rather than the precise mechanism of action. In this case, it may be more useful to consider the anatomical locus of anaesthetic action in the central nervous system and be satisfied with a less fundamental explanation of the mechanism which nevertheless may be more intelligible in terms of its effect upon the physiological function of the brain.

Physico-chemical theories of anaesthetic action will therefore only be considered rather briefly here and the demanding reader is referred to the excellent reviews by Smith and by Seeman.

Overton and Meyer were among the first to notice a correlation between lipid solubility and anaesthetic potency. However, lipid solubility is an important factor in gaining access to the brain or even to cell membranes. Ferguson correlated anaesthesia with thermodynamic activity but such molecular properties are related to other intrinsic physical properties of substances such as solubility, boiling point and molar refractivity, all of which show a high degree of correlation with anaesthesia.

Mullins proposed a critical volume theory from which has derived the idea that when anaesthetics dissolve in cell membranes they cause those membranes to expand. When the expansion reaches a critical point then normal membrane properties are so disrupted that anaesthesia ensues. That some anaesthetics do indeed alter the physico-chemical properties of membranes is shown by the fact that not only do they cause membrane expansion (at least in red blood cells) but they cause a disorganisation of membrane structure, as elegantly shown by the increased membrane fluidity in studies with nuclear magnetic resonance (NMR) techniques.

Other theories, such as those of Pauling, ascribe anaesthesia to interaction of anaesthetics with the aqueous phase of cell membranes, forming clathrates which alter membrane function. These clathrates may be stabilised by protein side chains in the physiological milieu.

Difficulties with physico-chemical theories

(1) Detailed studies of the effect of changes in pressure or temperature upon anaesthesia show that the effects are not always quite as predicted from the known effects of these factors on the clathrate formation. It is also difficult to account satisfactorily, in physico-chemical terms, for the fact that in a homologous series of anaesthetic compounds, the anaesthetic potency may increase in parallel with some physico-chemical characteristic up to a point beyond which the anaesthetic potency may decrease, whereas properties such as lipid solubility may continue to increase.

(2) It is difficult to understand why some substances should be anaesthetics, whereas very closely related substances, with rather similar physico-chemical characteristics should not only be lacking in anaesthetic action but in fact have quite the opposite effect on the central nervous system in causing convulsions. Examples of such opposing effects are shown in Fig. 6.3.

(3) Alphaxalone (Fig. 6.4) is a potent steroid anaesthetic, whereas the closely related Δ-16-alphaxalone not only lacks anaesthetic action but antagonises the effect of alphaxalone in isolated guinea pig cortex (Richards and Hesketh, 1975). Alphaxalone apparently does not change membrane fluidity, as measured by NMR, but it is not known whether Δ-16-alphaxalone antagonises the action of other anaesthetics. It is of course possible that the steroidal anaesthetics do indeed interact with specific membrane receptors, but this has yet to be demonstrated.

(4) Anaesthetics may depress other central nervous system functions in addition to consciousness. Thus, they may have

Anaesthetic   *Convulsant*

CF₃CHFBr   CF₃CH₂Br

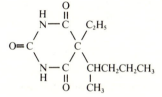

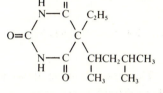

Pentobarbitone   5-ethyl-5-(1, 3-dimethylbutyl)
barbiturate

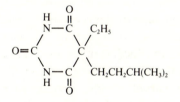

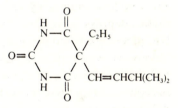

Amylobarbitone   5-ethyl-5-(8, 8 dimethylallyl)
barbiturate

Fig. 6.3. Closely related anaesthetics and convulsants.

analgesic actions, depress respiration or circulatory control. If they had only one action on the central nervous system then one would expect all agents to have similar relative potencies in all of these effects. Yet one finds that halothane has good analgesic properties but the barbiturates may have anti-analgesic actions; halothane depresses the blood pressure to a greater extent than does methoxy fluorane but the relative potencies are reversed for depression of respiration.

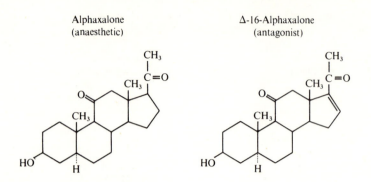

Fig. 6.4. Steroid anaesthetics.

There are no adequate explanations for these discrepancies but they should make one wary of accepting *in toto* any purely physico-chemical theory of anaesthetic action.

Localisation of the effects of anaesthetics on neurones

Pre- and postsynaptic effects. In sufficient concentrations, anaesthetics depress excitable cells in all parts of the nervous system, but effects are noted in some areas or on some parts of neurones at lower concentrations or earlier than effects at other sites. While a differential access of the anaesthetic to different parts of the nervous system may provide a partial explanation for such different sensitivities it is very unlikely that this factor predominates. It is more probable that some physiological functions or some neurones, are more affected by a quantitatively similar effect of the anaesthetic than are others.

For example, Weakly has shown pentobarbitone reduces the presynaptic release of transmitter responsible for the monosynaptic excitatory postsynaptic potential in motoneurones, even at subanaesthetic concentrations. However, he found, in agreement with others, that higher concentrations also caused a decrease in postsynaptic excitability.

Richards has examined the effects of a range of anaesthetics on pre- and postsynaptic phenomena in isolated cerebral cortex. Although all of the agents tested reduced the amplitude of evoked postsynaptic potentials they did not appear to do this by decreasing the electrical excitability of the postsynaptic membrane and there were differences between the agents, indicating that some anaesthetics (e.g. halothane) were acting to reduce the release of excitatory transmitter from the nerve terminals, whereas others (e.g. trichloroethylene) reduced the action of the transmitter on the postsynaptic membrane, as shown by the ability of trichlorethylene but not halothane to reduce the excitatory effect of glutamic acid.

Thus it may be concluded that general anaesthetics depress central neurones by effects on both pre- and postsynaptic mechanisms but the former are likely to be more susceptible with many agents. In very high concentrations the general anaesthetics may also depress nerve conduction, but this is not found at therapeutic concentrations.

Differential effects on excitatory neurotransmitters. A substance with a non-specific depressant action on cell membranes might be presumed to reduce the excitation of a particular neurone by any excitatory agent which is administered to it. It is therefore rather surprising to find that general anaesthetics selectively depress the excitation of cerebral cortical neurones by iontophoretically administered acetylcholine without reducing, but even enhancing, excitation by glutamic acid. The selective depression of excitation by acetylcholine is particularly pertinent to the question of anaesthesia because it is highly probable that cholinergic projections to the cerebral cortex are important in maintaining consciousness.

Krnjevic has noted that the effects of pentobarbitone on the membrane potential and resistance are similar to those of intracellularly injected calcium ions, which hyperpolarise the membrane and decrease resistance probably by increasing the membrane permeability to potassium ions. He has also shown that the probable mechanism of excitation of cortical neurones by acetylcholine is due to a reduction of the membrane permeability to potassium ions. It therefore seems likely that both anaesthetics and acetylcholine act on the same membrane permeability, but they have opposite effects.

A plausible explanation of the action of general anaesthetics which selectively reduce excitation by acetylcholine is that they reduce the sequestration of free internal calcium ions by brain mitochondria, so increasing the internal free calcium concentration and increasing permeability to potassium. Observations on the effects of anaesthetics on Ca^{2+} uptake by brain mitochondria are unfortunately few, but it is known that halothane at anaesthetic concentrations markedly reduces Ca^{2+} uptake by rat brain mitochondria.

The mechanism by which the sequestration of Ca^{2+} by mitochondria is suppressed by anaesthetics is unknown; it could be by a non-specific action on the mitochondrial membrane but it could also be due to a more specific effect on metabolic processes.

It is perhaps significant that the release of acetylcholine from the cerebral cortex, as measured by assay into a Perspex cup containing eserinised Ringer solution placed on the exposed surface of the cortex, is reduced by general anaesthetics and is higher in alert than in quiescent behavioural states. There may be several explanations for the reduction in release and the relative importance of each of these is not established. There is likely to be a direct depressant action of the anaesthetic on the release of the transmitter from presynaptic terminals but release would also be suppressed by any process which decreases the activity of the cholinergic neurones.

The cholinergic projection from the midbrain reticular formation is probably reduced in activity during anaesthesia, both by depressant effects on the projecting neurones themselves and by the reduction of afferent input to the cells during anaesthesia.

Effects on presynaptic inhibition. Presynaptic inhibition serves to reduce the release of transmitter from the central terminals of primary afferent nerve fibres and thereby reduces the flow of afferent information from peripheral receptors to the brain. Many general anaesthetics increase presynaptic inhibition, although the mechanism is obscure. They also increase a number of prolonged postsynaptic inhibitory processes in the brain and it may be significant that GABA is thought to be a common mediator of these effects.

A potentiation of inhibitory processes in the brain may therefore be supplementary to the other actions of general anaesthetics in causing a loss of consciousness.

Selective effects upon different areas of the brain and on spinal reflexes. It has long been known that general anaesthesia has a greater depressant effect upon polysynaptic spinal reflexes than upon monosynaptic reflexes. This may merely reflect the greater susceptibility of complex pathways to drug-induced depression. The same explanation may apply to the often-repeated demonstration that general anaesthetics tend to decrease activity in the reticular formation of the brain before effects can be detected elsewhere, although the selective effects upon cholinergic mechanisms may also be involved.

It was noted earlier that some inhibitory processes in the brain may be prolonged by general anaesthetics. However, Frank and Ohta have shown that the inhibition of spinal reflexes by stimulation of inhibitory regions of the reticular formation of the brain stem is reduced by concentrations of anaesthetics lower than those which block facilitation by stimulation of excitatory regions.

Conclusions. Even if general anaesthetics do act at the molecular level by a common non-specific action, and this seems by no means certain, then it is apparent that different neuronal membranes at different sites, including intracellular membranes, may be more susceptible than others. This may result from a particular membrane process being more important for the function of some cells than for others. In addition, different regions of the brain or even different pathways within the same area show differential susceptibilities to a given anaesthetic for reasons which are not entirely clear.

Anaesthesia, then, results from a depression of a number of functions of the brain and it is indeed fortunate that the selectivity of action results in a relatively selective depression of consciousness with minimal effects on some vital functions such as respiration and circulatory control. Such selectivity is clearly only marginal and the anaesthetics will depress all neuronal function in concentrations only slightly higher than those required for anaesthesia.

TOLERANCE TO ANAESTHETICS

Tolerance and physical dependence upon barbiturates may develop with continued use, although it is not so severe as with the opiates. This will clearly not be of great importance in the use of these agents as anaesthetics but will be more significant when they are used chronically as sedatives or hypnotics.

The tolerance depends upon the continuous presence of the agent and so is more evident with barbiturates which have a long half-life, such as phenobarbitone than with shorter-acting agents such as pentobarbitone. The tolerance seems to depend mainly upon neural adaptation to the continued presence of the drug, rather than to increased metabolism, because it has been clearly demonstrated that during the development of tolerance, sedative effects at the same blood level become progressively less. Tolerance may be produced by intravenous administration and so is not dependent upon changed absorption.

There is a cross-tolerance between the barbiturates and other classes of non-specific depressants of the nervous system (e.g. alcohol) but not with the opiates, indicating that in the latter case quite different mechanisms are involved.

Neural tolerance to the action of barbiturates has some significance in anaesthesia because it has been shown in rats that the brain level of barbital determined at the time of awakening is significantly increased after only five daily injections. In man, it has been shown that the plasma level of thiopentone at the time of awakening is about three times higher when sufficient thiopentone was given to produce anaesthesia lasting for about 5 h as compared with the level after a dose causing anaesthesia for only 1 h. The practical significance of such observations is that in order to obtain a prolonged anaesthesia with thiopentone, progressively higher plasma levels will need to be maintained which will increase the amount redistributing into fatty tissues and may lead to post-operative complications.

The mechanism of neural tolerance is completely unknown, but it may reasonably be assumed to represent homeostatic adaptation of the nervous system to the continued presence of the anaesthetic.

CHAPTER SEVEN

Pharmacological control of pain

PHYSIOLOGICAL BASIS

The sensation of pain is initiated in peripheral nociceptors by stimuli which are sufficiently intense to cause tissue damage. Perl has obtained evidence that at least some of the nociceptors respond only to painful stimuli: these nociceptive responses are conveyed to the central nervous system in Aδ fibres, but it is not unlikely that C fibre responses to painful stimuli may also be restricted to specific nociceptive fibres. It seems unlikely that pain sensation is evoked by intense activity in afferent fibres which normally convey other modality-specific information to the central nervous system, but nerve traffic in these fibres may well modify the sensation of pain evoked in nociceptive endings (Melzack, 1973). Tissue damage by intense stimuli leads to the liberation of physiologically active substances and so the pharmacology of the afferent nerve terminal is of some relevance to the actions of one group of pain-relieving drugs, the aspirin-like analgesics.

Upon entering the spinal cord pain fibres make extensive synaptic connections, particularly in the dorsal horn. Many nociceptive fibres cross in the anterior commissure and ascend the spinal cord in the lateral spinothalamic tracts. These fibres synapse extensively in reticular formation and thalamus and project diversely to cerebral cortex. It seems that many parts of the brain are involved in the sensation of pain and perhaps it is this factor which accounts for the complexity of the process. At all levels of the CNS it is probable that transmission of information relating to painful experience is modulated by modality-specific inputs. The pain experience may be crudely and rather arbitrarily separated into two components, the awareness of the painful stimulus and the affective reaction of the subject to that awareness. These two aspects of pain may be related to different parts of the CNS and in this respect it may be significant that the major group of analgesic drugs, the opiates, may have a greater effect on the subjective reaction to than on the awareness of a painful stimulus. In contrast to the aspirin-like analgesics, some of which act mainly at peripheral sites, the opiate (morphine-like) analgesics have no affect on peripheral components of pain but exert effects at all levels of the neuraxis.

ASPIRIN-LIKE DRUGS AND THE PERIPHERAL CONTROL OF PAIN

Aspirin-like drugs are usually taken by mouth and are relatively ineffective in severely painful conditions. However, they are quite effective in a large number of relatively minor painful conditions such as headache, neuralgia and pain arising from inflammatory conditions. Aspirin itself is the safest of the mild analgesics and the toxic reactions to this drug are rather mild. However, it may prolong bleeding time and cause minor gastric ulceration and haemorrhage, even with quite small doses. Mild intoxication or salicylism is characterised by headache, dizziness and confusion, problems with the visual and auditory systems, hyperventilation and disturbances of acid–base balance and various autonomic effects ranging from sweating and nausea to vomiting and diarrhoea. In more severe intoxication there may be grosser CNS disturbances including hallucinations and convulsions. Phenacetin and paracetamol (Fig. 7.1) are also usually well tolerated in therapeutic doses except for occasional skin rashes, but high levels may lead to methaemoglobinaemia and haemolytic anaemia or to potentially fatal hepatic and renal necrosis. Indomethacin and phenylbutazone are poorly tolerated in a relatively high proportion (up to 50%) of patients and are therefore not widely used. The most serious of these effects include thrombocytopenia, leukopenia, agranulocytosis and aplastic anaemia.

Mechanism of analgesia

The aspirin-like analgesics are all inhibitors of prostaglandin (PG) synthesis, although there are differences between the drugs in their

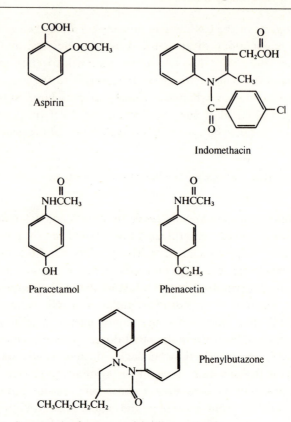

Fig. 7.1. Structures of some aspirin-like analgesics.

relative effectiveness on PG synthesis in different organs. The drugs display three important pharmacological actions, analgesia, anti-inflammatory effect and antipyretic action to varying degrees, and all of these actions can be attributed to inhibition of PG synthesis. Table 7.1 shows the relative analgesic and anti-inflammatory action of five of the drugs.

Two of the drugs, phenacetin and paracetamol, are analgesic but not anti-inflammatory and this has been correlated with an inability to inhibit PG synthesis in peripheral tissues although they are quite effective in the brain. It is therefore likely that the mechanism of analgesia may be comprised of both peripheral and central components varying in proportion from one drug to

Table 7.1. *Lack of correlation between analgesic and anti-inflammatory action of aspirin-like analgesics*

	Analgesic action	Anti-inflammatory action
Aspirin	+ +	+ +
Phenacetin	+ +	0
Paracetamol	+ +	0
Indomethacin	+ +[a]	+ + +
Phenylbutazone	+	+ + +

0, no action; +, + +, + + + refer to approximate order of potency.
[a] The analgesic effect of indomethacin may be the indirect consequence of anti-inflammatory action.

another. Undoubtedly the anti-inflammatory action contributes to the analgesic action by reducing the liberation of pain-producing substances in the vicinity of the peripheral nerve terminals but a direct effect on the mechanism of pain production has also been demonstrated.

The evidence that inhibition of PG synthesis is the mechanism of the anti-inflammatory effect is summarised below:

(*a*) Intradermal injections of PGE_1 or E_2 in rat or man causes hyperaemia and oedema.

(*b*) PGE_1 or E_2 is found in inflammatory exudates when carragenin is injected subcutaneously in rats.

(*c*) A mixture of PGs is found in the exudate in contact eczema in man.

(*d*) A reduction in the inflammatory response by drugs is accompanied by a reduction in the release of PGs.

The chief evidence for a peripheral action of aspirin on pain production derives from the work of Lim on dogs. He cross-perfused the spleen of a recipient dog with the blood from a donor animal.

It has long been known that bradykinin applied to the exposed blister base in man causes painful sensations and in animals it is known to activate the C fibres fairly selectively.

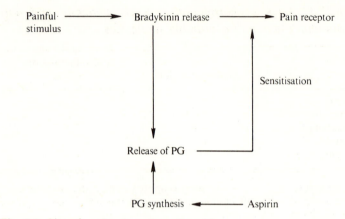

Fig. 7.2. Site of analgesic action of aspirin.

In the dog, the injection of bradykinin into the arterial supply of the spleen of the recipient dog caused discharges in the splenic nerve and signs of autonomic activation. Aspirin administered via the arterial supply of the recipient dog reduced the effect of the bradykinin, but failed to do so when injected into the systemic circulation. This demonstrates that aspirin was acting by a peripheral rather than by a central mechanism. In contrast, morphine failed to show such a peripheral action.

Bradykinin is known to release PGs from peripheral tissues. However, PGs themselves do not produce pain but sensitise nociceptors to the action of bradykinin, released by tissue-injury. Aspirin is thought to act by reducing the synthesis of prostaglandins, so reducing the sensitising action on released bradykinin (Fig. 7.2).

Paracetamol is a good analgesic which presumably acts by inhibition of PG synthesis at a central location but not peripherally. Aspirin also inhibits the synthetase from the brain and its anti-pyretic effect is undoubtedly due mainly to a central mechanism. It seems unreasonable therefore to suppose that the analgesic action of aspirin outlined above is the sole mechanism and it is more probable that in man the reduction in the stressful effects of pain is due to both central and peripheral components.

MORPHINE-LIKE DRUGS AND THE CENTRAL CONTROL OF
PAIN

The medical use of opium as a pain-relieving drug dates back at
least to the twelfth century and the use of soporofic sponges.
However, the absorption of morphine from the gastrointestinal
tract is unreliable and systemic administration, which avoids these
difficulties, was not possible until the active principle of opium had
been identified and the hypodermic syringe and needle had been
invented in the nineteenth century.

Opium may contain as much as 10% by weight of morphine and
0.5% of codeine, together with other alkaloids which are not
analgesic.

Structure of morphine-like drugs

Morphine, codeine and heroin are phenanthrene derivatives (Fig.
7.3) but this structure is not essential for analgesic activity. This
has become apparent from studies of the structure of a vast
number of analgesics which have been produced in an attempt,
largely unsuccessful, to avoid the abuse potential of the major
narcotic analgesics.

However, although pentazocine can cause addiction it is said
to be less addictive than the majority of opiates in equivalent
analgesic doses.

A common structure of analgesic drugs is not evident from
an examination of the two-dimensional structures (Fig. 7.3), but
many of them, e.g. methadone, are conformationally restricted
and, in three-dimensional models, closely resemble the shape of
the active D(-) isomer of morphine. Meperidine is less restricted,
but one of its several conformations corresponds to the D(-) isomer
of morphine.

Substitution of an allyl group on the nitrogen atom produces
compounds which are 'narcotic antagonists', i.e. they antagonise,
under suitable conditions, the analgesic, euphoric and respiratory
depressant effects of opiates and may precipitate withdrawal
symptoms in addicts. Some of these are partial agonists, e.g.
nalorphine which, when given alone, may produce the effects of

Analgesics

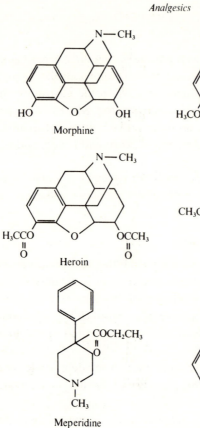

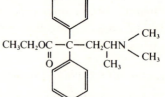

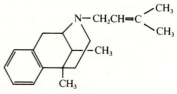

Antagonists

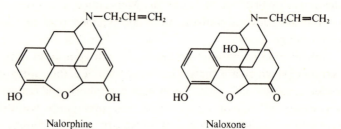

Fig. 7.3. Structures of some morphine-like drugs and antagonists.

morphine, including analgesia, but will counteract the action of morphine when the drugs are administered concurrently. The unpleasant psychological side-effects of nalorphine make it not only unlikely to cause dependence but also unacceptable as an analgesic in its own right. Pentazocine, however, has useful analgesic properties, while lacking the side-effects of nalorphine. Naloxone has relatively pure antagonistic actions, lacking many of the depressant actions of other antagonists.

Actions of morphine-like drugs

The most important medical use of opiates is as analgesics. They increase the tolerance to painful stimuli. They tend to subdue dull pain rather than sharp pain but this difference is largely dose-dependent. In some individuals, but not in others, the pain threshold is elevated. Although the painful stimulus is still perceived, the affective reaction to the pain is attenuated.

Euphoria is typical of most opiate analgesics and is probably the property that is most likely to lead to dependence. However, euphoria and sedation may also contribute to the analgesic effect and it is not yet clear to what extent the analgesic and euphoric actions are separable.

Opiates are also anxiety-reducing and may cause nausea and vomiting. The emetic effect is due to a stimulant action on the chemoreceptive trigger zone in the medulla and may be due to an action on dopamine receptors because apomorphine, an activator of dopamine receptors, is a powerful emetic. Morphine has also been shown to stimulate prostaglandin (PG) synthesis and both the increase in PG synthesis and the emetic effect is abolished by chlorpromazine, a dopamine antagonist (see Chapter 9). Thus it may be that morphine first activates dopamine receptors which leads to an increase in PG synthesis and then to the emetic action.

Morphine causes constipation by a spasmogenic action on the stomach and large and small intestines. This property is the basis of its early use in treating dysentery. It may cause biliary colic and severe epigastric pain due to a contraction of the sphincter of Oddi and the resulting increase in pressure in the bile ducts.

There are minimal effects on the cardiovascular system but the chief clinical hazard with opiates is a depression of respiratory exchange, evident even with therapeutic doses. Miosis is very characteristic of the morphine addict because tolerance to this action seems to be less marked than tolerance to many of the other effects. Morphine and codeine are also cough suppressants. The antitussive effect is not correlated with analgesia and drugs such as dextrorphan and noscapine are good antitussives but lack the analgesic and addictive properties of morphine.

Mechanism of action

The opiate receptor. Morphine and other drugs show high affinity, stereospecific binding to brain homogenates which correlates, with some exceptions, with the analgesic action. The exceptions, such as etorphine and codeine, can be satisfactorily explained on the basis of differences in lipid solubility, and therefore access to the brain, or enzymic degradation to more active products.

Localisation of the receptor. The receptor occurs in synaptic membranes although it is not yet known whether these are pre- or postsynaptic. The largest amount of receptor occurs in the anterior amygdala. The microinjection of morphine into this area of the brain does not cause analgesia and receptors in this area may be more related to the euphoric effect. However, the injection of morphine into the periaqueductal grey matter does cause analgesia and this area contains the second largest concentrations of receptor material. Areas of the brain concerned specifically with movement, e.g. cerebellum, contain rather low concentrations of opiate binding material.

Multiple conformations of the receptor. Pert and Snyder have shown that high concentrations of sodium inhibit the binding of opiate agonists but the affinity of pure antagonists is unchanged. They therefore suggest that there may be two configurations of the receptor, one of which selectively binds antagonists and the other agonists. They go even further to postulate that changes in the relative proportions of the two may be implicated in the development of tolerance but there is no direct evidence to

Endogenous	Tyr-Gly-Gly-Phe-Met
	Tyr-Gly-Gly-Phe-Leu
Synthetic	MeTyr-Gly-Gly-Phe-Met-CONH$_2$
	Tyr-D-Ala-Gly-Phe-Met-CONH$_2$

Fig. 7.4. Constitution of some enkephalins.

support such a contention. However, there is indirect evidence such as the fact that tolerant individuals show a reduced sensitivity to morphine but an increased sensitivity to antagonists.

Other evidence for multiple opiate receptors has been obtained from studies *in vitro* of the antagonism of leucine-enkephalin and naloxone binding to brain homogenate by morphine-like substances and polypeptides (Lord *et al.*, 1977). They have also demonstrated that there are differences in the relative potencies of a series of opiate agonists on a guinea pig ileum preparation and on the mouse vas deferens, and in the ability of naloxone to reverse the action of the agonists.

Endogenous morphine-like substances: the enkephalins. The enkephalins are endogenous morphine-like pentapeptides. Two, methionine enkephalin and leucine enkephalin (Fig. 7.4) have now been isolated from pig and bovine brain. The naturally occurring enkephalins are rapidly degraded by brain proteases, but synthetic derivatives are known which are resistant to proteolytic attack. Two of these are shown in Fig. 7.4: both have a terminal amide group.

The enkephalins have all of the actions of morphine and are analgesic when injected into the brain. β-endorphin, with thirty-one amino acid residues is also found in brain. It has analgesic properties and is highly concentrated in the anterior pituitary. It is not yet known whether the enkephalins or β-endorphin serve as neurotransmitters or modulators.

There is also evidence for a circulating morphine-like substance of low molecular weight (β-endorphin) which possibly originates from the pituitary because it disappears after hypophysectomy. Such substances may be implicated in the mechanism of acupuncture analgesia because, both experimentally and in man, electro-acupuncture effects are antagonised by the opiate antagonist naloxone. β-endorphin (or a similar polypeptide) has also been shown to be released in conditions of stress.

It was originally thought that the enkephalins might lead to a new series of non-addicting analgesics. However, tolerance to the action of enkephalins does develop and it seems unlikely that a non-addicting analgesic could be developed from such substances, even though an orally active enkephalin with analgesic activity has been synthesised.

Consequences of activation of opiate receptors. It has long been known that morphine blocks the electrically evoked contractions of guinea ilea and reduces the release of acetylcholine. These effects have a remarkable parallel to the analgesic actions and to binding to opiate receptors both in brain and intestine. The effects of morphine are also mimicked by the enkephalins and are probably not restricted to cholinergic neurones because there is also a block of the release of catecholamines.

Opiates reduce the release of acetylcholine from the surface of the cerebral cortex. This effect is less in animals made tolerant and is antagonised by naloxone. However, the effect is probably exerted subcortically because it is only produced with systemic injection and not with local application to the cortex.

Morphine blocks the evoked release of substance P from slices of rat trigeminal nucleus. This indicates that the polypeptide, substance P, may also play a role in analgesia, particularly when considered in relation to the fact that injections of substance P itself into the brain is reported to produce analgesia.

There have been many neuropharmacological and neurophysiological studies on the site of action of morphine in the brain. Microinjection into the periaqueductal grey causes anaesthesia and supraspinal effects are undoubtedly of prime importance. However, morphine blocks ascending pain pathways by a direct depressant action on nociceptive spinal neurones, by modifying the descending, supraspinal, control of these spinal neurones and possibly also by an excitatory action on non-nociceptive cells, so 'closing the gate' in terms of the 'gate theory' of Melzack and Wall.

Tolerance and dependence

Tolerance and dependence are very marked in opiate drugs compared with the much weaker effects in the general depressants. In man, an initial dose of 100–200 mg of morphine could lead to very severe depression and may even be fatal. In tolerant individuals even 4 g may have no adverse effects. The addict may therefore ultimately require enormous quantities of the drug in order to maintain the habit. Thus, in addition to the physical debilitation caused by the drug itself, there is also the social disintegration caused by the need for ever-increasing financial requirements to purchase ever-increasing quantities of illicit drugs.

The habit is self-reinforcing, as shown in behavioural experiments in monkeys. The animals were able to self-administer intravenous injections of morphine by pressing a lever. Over a period of several days the daily intake of morphine gradually increased to a stable level of about 100 mg/kg/day. Other activities, such as eating, drinking and sex were partly ignored. In addition to the self-reinforcement the habit is probably maintained by the need to avoid withdrawal symptoms.

The time course of the development of tolerance is extremely rapid.

In studies in post-addicts it has been shown that tolerance to morphine is evident after just one day of treatment (heroin is similar) and increases progressively and rapidly over a period of weeks.

Cross-tolerance between opiates is quite characteristic but does not extend to general depressant drugs such as the barbiturates or alcohol.

Tolerance depends upon maintaining high plasma levels of the drug. Therefore a temporary withdrawal of the drug will reduce the level of tolerance and so reduce the requirement for large quantities of drug. A sudden reduction of plasma levels or the injection of an antagonist leads to physical withdrawal symptoms, including restlessness and craving, lachrimation, perspiration, chills, fever, vomiting, panting, aches and pains, dilatation of the pupil and piloerection ('cold-turkey'). The withdrawal symptoms reach a maximum about 2 days after withdrawing morphine, but are slower in onset and less marked with methadone. This is the basis for methadone substitution therapy and is dependent on the relative plasma half-lives of morphine and methadone.

Mechanism of tolerance and dependence. Tolerance is not due to decreased absorption, penetration into the brain or decreased plasma half-life, nor is it due to an increased non-specific binding.

The progressive onset suggests that the mechanism is a slowly adapting one. To a large degree, the tolerance is likely to be due to compensatory homeostatic mechanisms coming into play, which counteract the drug effect. However, there may also be compensatory mechanisms occurring at the synaptic level, such as changes in drug–receptor interactions, number of receptors or their configuration or changes in transmitter turnover and release.

CHAPTER EIGHT

Drugs and disorders of movement

PHYSIOLOGICAL BASIS

Movement of the limbs is brought about by the coordinated contractions of synergistic muscles with reciprocal relaxation of some antagonists. The overall pattern of movement is directly related to the patterns of activation and inhibition of the spinal α-motoneurones. These patterns are established by the basic 'wiring' of the CNS and by the flexibility of the functional connections established by integrated control over transmission in the neuronal circuits.

The patterns of activation and inhibition of spinal motoneurones and changes from moment to moment are controlled by a hierarchical series of modulating systems involving all levels of the CNS. The operation of feedback loops, in which the output of the control system, or of movement itself, is continuously monitored and utilised to modify the following sequence of events so as to establish a predictable course of events, with minimal interference from extraneous disturbances. Superimposed on all of these systems is volitional control, presumably involving the highest levels of the CNS, which can initiate, modulate or arrest a particular sequence.

Our knowledge of the system derives from the many advances made in the realms of neurophysiology, biochemistry, anatomy and pathology. It must, however, be admitted that although the operation of parts of the system have been worked out in considerable detail, our comprehension of the exact integration of each subsystem with another is rather rudimentary.

The establishment of the basic patterns of excitation and inhibition of spinal motoneurones, and, consequently of the basic patterns of movement, are largely attributable to coordination established at the spinal level. The muscle spindle receptors play a paramount role in this control. They not only operate as a negative feedback, continuously adjusting motor output to suit the demands of the moment, but are also involved in the indirect activation of α-motoneurones through the gamma-loop. Thus, it has been established that volitional movement usually involves the simultaneous activation of both the α-motoneurones innervating the extrafusal muscle fibres and the γ-motoneurones innervating intrafusal fibres. The spinal reflexes set up by impulses in spindle afferent fibres (Group IA and II) are organised in a reciprocal fashion to cause appropriate excitation or inhibition of flexor or extensor motoneurones. In addition, the receptors in the tendon organs, giving rise to IB afferent fibres, receptors in joints and in the skin and recurrent inhibition via the Renshaw cell also play a role in the integration of muscle contraction at the spinal level by postsynaptic excitatory and pre- or postsynaptic inhibitory mechanisms.

The input to the CNS from peripheral receptors is relayed to supraspinal control centres via the ascending tracts of the spinal cord by lemniscal and extra-lemniscal paths. The patterns set up at the spinal level are then modulated by a complexity of control signals in the descending motor tracts.

There are three, relatively large, parts of the brain which are outstanding for their particular ability to influence movement. These are the cerebellum, basal ganglia and somatosensory and motor areas of the cerebral cortex. Of these, the detailed operation of the cerebellum is perhaps best understood. The reasons for this are probably attributable to the beautifully geometric organisation of its neurones, which renders it particularly amenable to neurophysiological investigation. The sole output via the Purkinje cell axons is inhibitory to the deep cerebellar nuclei and the major input is via climbing or mossy fibres. The neurones of the cerebellum and cerebellar nuclei are involved in a delicately arranged series of feed-forward and feedback loops which integrate and coordinate a wide variety of information from peripheral receptors and other brain structures. The cerebellum is thought to be involved in the acquisition and learning of complex motor tasks, so that it may execute pre-programmed sequences of movements in a precise fashion with minimal regulation from other brain areas.

The basal ganglia, comprising mainly the caudate nucleus, putamen and globus pallidus, together with the substantia nigra seems to be primarily involved in movement control and is often involved in disorders of movement. Its precise functions are incompletely understood and the concepts regarding its place in the hierarchical control system are largely derived from observations made in pathological conditions. Nevertheless, it is clear that many disorders in which there are involuntary or abnormal movements or defects in the ability to initiate or arrest patterns of movement seem to have a basis in malfunctions in the basal ganglia. Neurophysiological and anatomical studies have demonstrated the occurrence of numerous feedback loops within the system and in its connections to cerebral cortex.

By convention, the cerebral cortex is usually considered to represent the highest level of volitional control over motor systems. However, its potential cannot be realised without the cooperation of the subordinate control systems in the basal ganglia and cerebellum which are probably the encoders of 'command' signals from cortex into the complex, integrated patterns of movement which are so evident in the normal individual. Although direct cortico-spinal fibres may have effects at the spinal level, destruction of the pyramidal tracts leads to relatively minor motor deficits limited mainly to very fine volitional movements, particularly of the digits. It must therefore be concluded that the major control signals for movement and posture leave the brain by extrapyramidal systems of nerve fibres.

TYPES OF MOVEMENT DISORDERS

Disorders of movement control can exhibit a wide variety of symptoms which form the basis for diagnosis. They can be produced by a variety of causes including trauma, infection and lesions of unknown origin. Some examples are given below.

Metabolic deficiency. In the chronic alcoholic, there may be a polyneuritis which may in part be due to a metabolic or vitamin deficiency. In advanced stages of the disease (Korsakoff's syndrome) there may be confusion, loss of memory and cerebellar degeneration.

Phenylketonuria is a disease produced by an inborn error in the metabolism of phenylalanine to tyrosine and is accompanied by high levels of abnormal phenylketones in the urine. This may be accompanied by mental retardation and siezures which, unless treated early in life by a reduction in dietary phenylalanine, may lead to permanent deficits.

Down's syndrome (mongolism) is primarily an inherited degenerative disease of the CNS causing mental defectiveness, but is also accompanied by a hypotonia of skeletal muscle. It is possible that this is related to a defect in the metabolism of 5-hydroxytryptamine because administration of the precursor, 5-hydroxytryptophan may reduce the hypotonia.

Infection. Examples of disorders of movement caused by infections of the CNS include neurosyphilis, poliomyelitis and post encephalitic Parkinson's disease. In neurosyphilis the invading spirochaete causes a destruction of dorsal column fibres leading to a mild to severe ataxia and, in a low proportion of untreated infections, to a more severe form of dementia paralytica. The only treatment available is to use penicillin, to destroy the invading spirochaete. Poliomyelitis is due to a viral infection causing destruction of anterior horn cells and flaccid paralysis. There is no effective treatment except for the prophylactic use of vaccines.

Drugs and toxic substances. Many drugs may cause disorders of movement as a consequence of their central actions. Notorious among these are the phenothiazine and butyrophenone antipsychotic agents. Such drugs interfere with function and do not generally cause permanent lesions. They are therefore reversible. In contrast, a number of heavy metals including copper, arsenic, lead and manganese can cause permanent, degenerative lesions in the CNS. Toxins, such as tetanus toxin, may cause slowly reversible motor dysfunction by interfering with specific transmitter mechanisms.

Miscellaneous and unknown causes. Examples of such disorders which will later be considered in more detail are epilepsy, spasticity and cerebral palsy and idiopathic Parkinson's disease.

Hereditary mechanisms. We have already briefly considered the occurrence of hypotonia in mongolism. Huntington's chorea is an inherited basal ganglia disease which will later be considered in more detail.

In many of these disorders, e.g. spasticity and Parkinson's disease, the occurrence of visible symptoms has often been preceded by degenerative CNS lesions, either discrete or widespread. Such pathological changes are permanent and cannot be reversed by treatment. Drug treatment is therefore palliative, producing a regression of symptoms but rarely a cure.

DRUG ACTIONS

Convulsants

Several, but not all, convulsant agents act by specifically interfering with amino acid inhibitory transmission in the CNS. The structure of strychnine, picrotoxin and bicuculline is given in Fig. 8.1.

Strychnine. This causes tonic contractions of all limb muscles, including extensor and flexor muscles. The limbs are usually tonically extended due to the more powerful contractions of the antigravity muscles which in most species are extensor.

It was shown long ago that strychnine caused a block of spinal postsynaptic inhibitory mechanisms and it has been more recently demonstrated that it does so by competing with the spinal inhibitory transmitter, glycine, for its receptor sites on postsynaptic membranes. Strychnine binding to brain fractions has been employed to study the distribution of glycine receptors and antagonism of inhibition by strychnine is indicative that glycine is the inhibitory transmitter. Strychnine has been shown to block many types of spinal postsynaptic inhibition including recurrent,

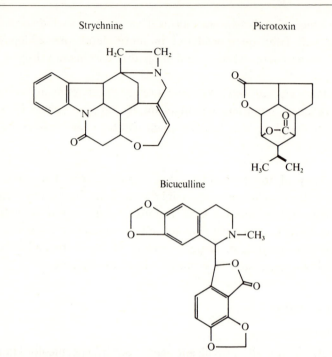

Fig. 8.1. Structures of some convulsant agents.

Renshaw cell inhibition, reciprocal IA inhibition, inhibition produced by stimulation of IB afferent fibres from Golgi tendon organs and some reticulospinal inhibitions. Antagonism to post-synaptic inhibition has also been demonstrated in the cuneate nucleus and medial geniculate nucleus, but, in general, supraspinal inhibition is not antagonised by strychnine.

When applied topically to the cerebral cortex, strychnine causes electrical seizure activity but the mechanism of this effect is uncertain.

Picrotoxin and bicuculline. These agents also cause convulsions but the convulsions are clonic in nature, with alternating periods of extension and flexion of the limbs. The mechanism is quite different from that of strychnine. Both agents are ineffective against the inhibitory effect of iontophoretically administered glycine but they both block the inhibitory effects of GABA at spinal and supraspinal sites. GABA is thought to be the mediator of presynaptic inhibition in the spinal cord and of postsynaptic inhibition at many supraspinal synaptic junctions. Antagonism of synaptically evoked inhibition by either of these agents is there-fore indicative that GABA is the inhibitory transmitter, particu-larly if it can be shown that the amino acid is released on activation of the synapses.

Tetanus toxin. Tetanus toxin is liberated by *clostridium tetani*, which is a normal inhabitant of the gut of horses and sheep. The bacillus is an anaerobic organism which flourishes in deep, penetrating wounds. The toxin is transported into the CNS from the site of primary infection along sensory and motor nerves and may then spread slowly through the CNS giving rise to local and then generalised convulsions.

Like strychnine, tetanus toxin blocks spinal inhibitions with no effect on excitatory transmission. However, the toxin does not antagonise the inhibitory actions of locally administered glycine or GABA and acts by reducing the release of these amino acids from presynaptic terminals. It has no effects on the levels of the amino acids in spinal cord. It is not known whether the toxin affects the release of other inhibitory transmitter agents.

Anti-epileptic agents

Epilepsy may be produced in many ways. It may be caused by infection, trauma, tumours, etc., but often the causative factor is unidentified. It may be broadly classified into two types. Focal seizures are initiated at a specific locus in the brain, usually in a cerebral hemisphere. Typical seizure activity first appears at this locus and there may be abnormal EEG activity in this region, even during the interictal periods. Seizure activity may then spread, gradually involving larger areas of first the ipsilateral and then the contralateral cortex and leads finally to generalised convulsions as in grand mal seizures.

The initial symptoms of an impending epileptic convulsion, the 'aura', depend upon the site of the primary focus. If the aura is associated with localised sensory or motor phenomena, then the focus is likely to be in the somatosensory or motor cortex of the opposite side. Visual phenomena may be associated with a focus in the occipital cortex. If the initial symptoms consist of a loss of consciousness then the focus may be in the frontal lobes.

Psychomotor epilepsy is another form of focal epilepsy which has a locus in the temporal lobes, and drug treatment may differ from that used in grand mal.

Centrencephalic seizures in petit mal are not accompanied by a preliminary aura. The EEG shows a characteristic pattern with a typical 3-per-second rhythm. Interictal discharges are rare. The first symptoms may be a sudden loss of consciousness which is usually brief, lasting for only a few seconds, and is often unaccompanied by muscle movements. The seizure is bilateral and is probably initiated in a midline structure of the brain.

Drug treatment depends upon the type of epilepsy, and accurate diagnosis is important because the wrong drug may make the condition worse rather than better.

Bromides were introduced in the last century for the treatment of epilepsy and were, for many years, the only effective treatment available. Their use has now been discontinued because of severe toxic side-effects, tolerable in the absence of any other treatment, but no longer acceptable since less toxic and more effective drugs are now available. Some of the more modern drugs are listed in Table 8.1.

In the severe, repeated convulsions of status epilepticus, anticonvulsants, sedatives or anaesthetics of various types may be used, e.g. barbiturates, diphenylhydantoin, benzodiazepines.

The mode of action of anti-epileptic agents is not very clear. Little is known of the action of drugs utilised in petit mal. However, phenobarbitone and diphenylhydantoin decrease post-tetanic potentiation in the CNS and this may be the basis of the effect in preventing the spread of seizure activity. At high sodium:potassium ratios *in vitro*, diphenylhydantoin activates the sodium–potassium-activated ATPase in synaptosomes but this does not occur at low sodium:potassium ratios. It also increases sodium transport in intestinal mucosa. It could act either by

Table 8.1. *Anti-epileptic drugs*

Type of seizure	Drugs used
Focal (grand mal)	Phenobarbitone, mephobarbitone, diphenylhydantoin, primidone, mephenytoin
Focal (temporal lobe)	Diphenylhydantoin, mephanytoin, primidone, phenacemide
Centrencephalic (petit mal)	Trimethadione, paramethadione, phensuximide, ethosuximide

blocking sodium channels or by decreasing calcium ion permeability, but this remains to be established.

Spasticity

Spasticity is a muscle rigidity of central origin. Muscle spasm may also have a basis in peripheral phenomena, often involving painful conditions, e.g. arthritic spasm, migraine or trauma, but the treatment is quite different.

Spasticity of CNS origin may give rise to distorted postures or movements and is not usually accompanied by pain. It may be produced by a myriad of CNS lesions ranging from those involving spinal tracts to more extensive lesions in the brain. The symptoms are varied according to the site of the lesion and may range from overactivity to immobility and are considered to be extrapyramidal. Typically, stretch reflexes are exaggerated, e.g. the Babinski sign.

Spasticity is often aggravated by anxiety and many of the drugs used with moderate success in the treatment of spasticity are anxiety-reducing agents.

Spasticity may be extremely marked in cerebral palsy in children, in which there may be widespread brain lesions giving rise to mental defectiveness and motor disorders.

Curare-like agents have been used by the parenteral route to reduce spasticity in particularly severe or acute episodes, but they are highly dangerous and are not widely employed.

The centrally acting muscle relaxants have been more widely employed, but with varying degrees of success, possibly due to different selection procedures employed. In general, it may be said that these drugs may have some beneficial effects in some patients but the improvement is not dramatic. More effective drugs are required.

The centrally acting muscle relaxants include mephanesin, meprobamate, carisoprodal, librium and valium and a new antispastic drug, β-chlorophenyl-GABA (Lioresal).

Most of these drugs differentially reduce polysynaptic reflexes in experimental animals, leaving monosynaptic reflexes such as the 'knee-jerk' relatively unchanged. It is therefore considered that they reduce transmission through chains of interneurones, the longer the chain the greater the susceptibility to the drug, and they have therefore sometimes been called 'interneuronal blocking' agents.

The wide variety of drugs which share this property indicates that they may not all act in the same way at the cellular level. Little is known about the basic mechanisms by which they produce muscle relaxation but some of their properties will be considered later in the chapter on anxiety-reducing drugs.

Wilson's disease, Huntington's chorea and Parkinson's disease

Disorders of the group of brain nuclei known collectively as the basal ganglia give rise to a number of motor symptoms including a paucity of movement (akinesia), rigidity of movement, involuntary movements such as chorea, hemiballism or athetosis and tremors. The disorders selected for consideration here are those in which there is some knowledge of the basic disorders and of the mechanisms by which drugs produce their beneficial effects.

Wilson's disease. In Wilson's disease there are clear lesions of the putamen and globus pallidus which together represent the lenticular nucleus. There are also lesions in the liver giving rise to the term hepatolenticular disease. When the condition arises early in life the chief symptom may be rigidity, but later in life the symptoms are mainly athetosis and chorea.

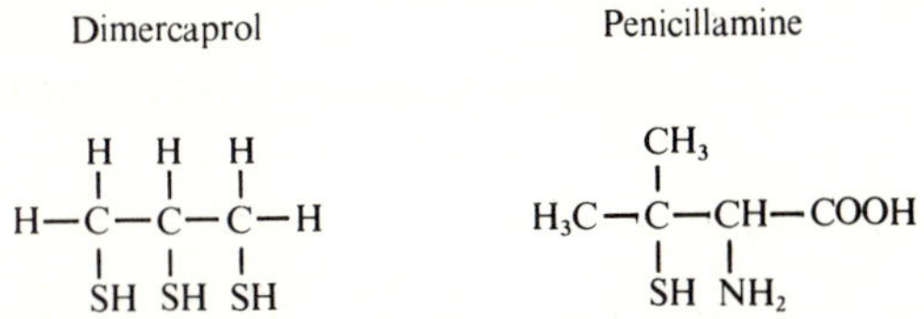

Dimercaprol   Penicillamine

```
    H   H   H                      CH₃
    |   |   |                      |
H—C—C—C—H              H₃C—C—CH—COOH
    |   |   |                      |   |
   SH  SH  SH                     SH  NH₂
```

Fig. 8.2. Copper chelators.

The lesions are caused by the localised accumulation of copper, which is toxic to neurones. Normally, plasma copper ions are chelated by ceruloplasmin, which is deficient in Wilson's disease. Treatment consists of the administration of copper-chelating agents coupled with a reduction in dietary copper.

The first drug of this type to be used was dimercaprol (British Anti-Lewisite), developed as an antidote to arsenical poisoning. However, a more modern drug, penicillamine, is less toxic (Fig. 8.2).

Huntington's chorea (*senile chorea*). Huntington's chorea is a hereditary disease of the basal ganglia and cerebral cortex. Choreiform movements and mental deterioration occur in adult life and are accompanied by widespread lesions in the brain, especially in the caudate and lenticular nuclei. The disease occurs in both sexes of all races and only rarely does it miss a generation. Symptoms usually occur between the ages of 30 and 50 and may be increased by emotional disturbance and by voluntary movements but tend to disappear during sleep. Chorea is increased by treatment with L-DOPA, which may precipitate symptoms in siblings in whom there was no other evidence of the disease.

Recent biochemical studies of post-mortem specimens have shown no defect in the level of dopamine in the brain. However, there is a deficiency in the caudate nucleus of glutamic acid decarboxylase, the enzyme principally involved in the synthesis of the inhibitory transmitter, GABA, which is probably associated with a 'GABA-projection' from caudate nucleus to substantia nigra. In some, but not all, brains there is also a decrease in the

1. *Parkinson's disease*

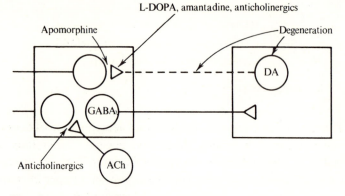

2. *Huntington's chorea*

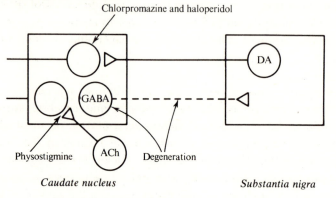

Fig. 8.3. Drug action in the basal ganglia.

content of choline acetyl transferase which is associated with cholinergic projections to the caudate nucleus. The reduction in choline acetyl transferase may also be associated with a reduction in the amount of cholinergic receptors. Since the reduction of cholinergic receptor is not always accompanied by a reduction in the level of the synthesising enzyme, it has been postulated that a postsynaptic lesion may precede the presynaptic change.

Haloperidol ahd chlorpromazine are useful therapeutically. Since these substances are dopamine receptor antagonists (see chapter on antischizophrenic drugs) and have no marked effects on either cholinergic or GABA-mediated transmission, it is possible that they produce their beneficial effect by partially restoring a functional balance between dopaminergic transmission and cholinergic and gabanergic transmission in the basal ganglia, rather than by a direct restitution of the deranged function in the cholinergic and gabanergic systems (see Fig. 8.3).

Haloperidol has also been used in treating the syndrome of Gilles de la Tourette, characterised by bizarre tics, coprolalia and convulsions and the absence of a family history of the disease. However, nothing is known of the mechanisms involved in this syndrome.

There is also a report that the anticholinesterase substance physostigmine decreased the involuntary movements in patients with Huntington's chorea. This would fit well with the postulated defect in cholinergic transmission but the anticholinesterase drugs are unlikely to be very acceptable due to the overactivity of peripheral cholinergic systems.

Parkinson's disease. Serendipity has played a large part in the discovery of new drugs, particularly those used in the treatment of disorders of the CNS. The use of L-dihydroxyphenylalanine (L-DOPA) in Parkinsonism is an exceptional example of a successful, rational approach to treatment which probably would not have occurred without the simultaneous development of knowledge of central neurotransmitter mechanisms, coupled with basic pharmacological and biochemical observations and an understanding of the underlying pathology.

The disease was first described in 1817 by James Parkinson and can be considered to be of three types: (i) symptomatic; (ii) postencephalitic; (iii) idiopathic.

The symptoms are similar, but not necessarily identical, in all types of the disease and consist of tremors, which tend to disappear during volitional movement, poverty of movement (akinesia), including difficulties in initiating or arresting a movement or sequence of movements, impairment of handwriting (micrographia), stooped, stiff postures, impaired speech and therefore difficulties in communication and 'cog-wheel' rigidity. However, mental faculties are not generally impaired.

Symptomatic Parkinson's disease may follow injury to the CNS caused by trauma, senile arteriosclerosis, carbon monoxide poisoning, manganese and other metallic poisoning. In all such instances, the lesions produced may be irreversible. Some drugs, in particular the phenothiazine and butyrophenone antipsychotic drugs, which are dopamine-receptor antagonists, also produce some of the symptoms of the disease.

Postencephalitic Parkinson's disease was first observed as a consequence of an epidemic of a disease of unknown aetiology called encephalitis lethargica in 1916–17. There have been no later known occurrences of this disease. The neurological signs of the basal ganglia disorder occurred some years later, but occasionally even in young children. In contrast, idiopathic Parkinson's disease is of unknown origin and rarely occurs before the age of 40 and reaches a peak between the ages of 50 and 60 years. The incidence has been estimated to be as high as 1:40 in some studies but in others it was 1:500. Genetic factors are not clearly defined although males are more prone to the disease than females. There is usually a progressive deterioration over a 10–15 year time span from the onset of symptoms and the time course is not greatly affected by symptomatic drug treatment.

One of the first indications in the 1950s that there might be a deficiency of catecholamine transmission in the brain in Parkinson's disease arose from the observation that reserpine, known to cause a depletion of brain catecholamines, caused akinesia in man and that these effects could be counteracted by treatment with L-DOPA. A little later it was shown that dopamine was highly concentrated in the basal ganglia and, shortly, thereafter, that the concentration in the basal ganglia was very low in the brains of patients who had died from the disease. The studies with fluorescence techniques in experimental animals later established the presence of the dopaminergic projection from the substantia nigra to the neo-striatum.

The initial trials with L- and DL-DOPA in Parkinson's disease did not meet with a great deal of success, either because of the deterrent effect of toxic actions or because the amount administered was too small. In 1967, it was found that large amounts (3–8 g/day by mouth) of L-DOPA produced a remarkable improvement in the akinesia and rigidity, with less effect on tremors. However, side-effects are numerous but, fortunately, only the psychic side-effects, seen in only about 10% of the patients, are usually sufficient to necessitate withdrawal of the drug. Other side-effects, such as involuntary movements of athetosis or chorea, and postural hypotension are more numerous and may limit the maximum amount of drug that can be administered but are generally not severe enough to warrant removal of the drug. Gastrointestinal effects are extremely common, particularly during the early stages of treatment, but can be reduced by the simultaneous administration of a peripheral DOPA-decarboxylase inhibitor such as carbidopa. The reduction of a peripheral decarboxylation allows more L-DOPA to enter the CNS, with a consequent reduction in dose, but this does not reduce the incidence of central side-effects.

Treatment with L-DOPA is essentially replacement therapy, in which deficient functioning of the dopaminergic system is partially restored by increasing the availability of precursor to the remaining functional dopamine-containing terminals in the striatum. However, it is not certain that some decarboxylation of L-DOPA to dopamine does not occur elsewhere, for example, in 5-hydroxytryptamine-containing neurones.

Belladonna alkaloids were first used by Charcot in 1892 to treat patients with Parkinson's disease. Later, the *synthetic anticholinergic drugs* such as atropine, benztropine, trihexyphenidyl (Artane) were introduced up to 1947. In 1948 the antihistamine, diphenhydramine was employed with some success but not all antihistamine compounds are effective in Parkinson's disease. Developed from the antihistaminic phenothiazine compound, promethazine, which is of no value in treating Parkinson's disease, other anticholinergic phenothiazines such as ethopropazine and diethazine were introduced as anti-Parkinsonian agents.

None of these drugs are as effective as L-DOPA but they may be used synergistically with L-DOPA so as to reduce the incidence of side-effects.

The anticholinergic agents have a variety of pharmacological actions which may contribute to their therapeutic effect. First, the

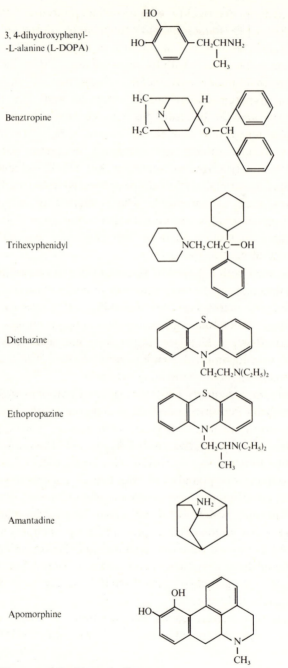

3, 4-dihydroxyphenyl-
-L-alanine (L-DOPA)

Benztropine

Trihexyphenidyl

Diethazine

Ethopropazine

Amantadine

Apomorphine

Fig. 8.4. Drugs and Parkinson's disease.

anticholinergic action *per se* may block cholinergic projections to the striatum, so restoring the balance between cholinergic and dopaminergic projections to this structure. Secondly, they have been shown to block the uptake of DA by brain synaptosomes *in vitro*. This may increase the amount of dopamine available to produce an effect on postsynaptic receptors. Finally, the drugs cause the release of newly synthesised dopamine in the striatum and so may facilitate transmission.

Amantadine was originally introduced as an antiviral agent but was subsequently found to have a limited use in treating patients with Parkinson's disease. It also has an effect on the dopamine system to release the transmitter.

Apomorphine is best known for its emetic effect but has a minor therapeutic effect in Parkinson's disease. Its major interest is in the fact that it reduces the turnover of dopamine in the brain, shown by a reduction in the production of the metabolite homovanillic acid. It has been suggested that apomorphine directly activates postsynaptic dopamine receptors and regulates dopamine turnover by a negative-feedback pathway from post-synaptic neurones to the dopaminergic neurones in the substantia nigra. This feedback loop may involve the striato-nigral GABA pathway mentioned earlier.

Fig. 8.4 shows the structures of some drugs which are effective in Parkinson's disease and Fig. 8.3 summarises the possible mechanisms of action. It will be seen that all drugs influence the dopamine system to some extent but that some, notably the anticholinergic drugs, also have other actions.

CHAPTER NINE

Drugs and mental disorders

INTRODUCTION

Drugs have been used from time immemorial to change mood or perception but only in recent times has there been any great advance in the systematic use of chemical agents for the treatment of mental disorders. The success of psychotropic drug therapy may be judged by the completely changed nature of psychiatric hospitals and in the treatment which they afford and in the ability of many patients to resume at least some degree of operation, even if often restricted, within the society at large.

Despite the therapeutic success of psychotherapeutic agents, we are only just beginning to unravel the mysteries of the mechanisms by which they act and, on the whole, still have no clear ideas about the basic defects which cause malfunction. In part, this can be attributed to the very complexity of human behaviour and therefore in the manner in which abnormalities may be manifest. Even the definition of what constitutes abnormal behaviour is dependent upon time and place, but within a given society gross disturbances in behaviour will be clearly discernable. Nevertheless, there will be occasions when the decision to treat what is judged to be abnormal behaviour poses ethical, as well as medical, problems. In general, treatment may be indicated when the behavioural disturbance is associated with an inability of the patient to continue with his normal role and position in society, to the detriment either of his personal circumstances or, in extreme cases, to the society in which he operates.

Psychotropic drugs may be divided into several categories, on the basis of the characterisation of the disorders for which they are most used. Anxiety states are characteristic of psychoneurotic conditions in which anxiety, a normal component of behaviour, is exaggerated to the point at which the patient is no longer able to cope with the normal ups and downs of everyday living. In such conditions anxiety-reducing drugs such as the barbiturates, and minor tranquillisers, e.g. meprobamate and the benzodiazepines, have made a considerable impact. It may even be argued that they have become so well accepted by both the medical profession and society that they are greatly overused as universal panaceas in conditions in which it would be far better if the patient learned to cope with or find practical solutions to his problems, rather than attempting to find escape from them.

Psychotic disorders are more severe and may progress to incapacitating mental illness characterised by grossly abnormal mood, emotional behaviour and a loss of contact with reality, including delusions and hallucinations. Although such disorders are commonly attributed to organic changes, the nature of the defects are virtually unknown. Undoubtedly, hereditary, socio-logical and environmental factors, besides organic or biochemical defects may all contribute to varying degrees in the manifestation of the disorder and in the likely success of treatment. There are two major classes of drugs which have proved to be of immense value in the management of psychotic behaviour. Major tran-quillisers like chlorpromazine, the first really useful drug of its type which is still probably used more than any other, and others such as the butyrophenones and dibenzazepines are used in the management of schizophrenia. Antidepressants, and in particular the tricyclic antidepressants, are used in the treatment of affective disorders displaying a marked and incapacitating de-pressive component whereas lithium salts are used in the long term control of manic depression.

Although there is little evidence that the drugs directly affect a disordered process, the fact that they alleviate symptoms is in itself desirable and may create an internal environment in which progress towards rectifying personality changes are made possible by interrupting the vicious circle in which the disturbed behaviour affects social interactions which in turn leads to a further deterioration in behaviour.

Other drugs such as LSD or mescaline may cause behavioural and perceptual disturbances but it is doubtful whether they are of any therapeutic value, despite some claims to the contrary.

However, they are of interest because the disturbances which they produce have some resemblance to schizophrenic symptoms and a study of the mechanisms by which they act may provide some insight into the basic psychotic disorder.

ANXIETY-REDUCING DRUGS

The drugs used to relieve psychoneurotic anxiety are frequently sedative and hypnotic. Some are also anticonvulsant. Many drugs have been examined both experimentally and clinically but those most frequently used fall into three classes: the barbiturates, e.g. amylobarbitone and phenobarbitone; the propanediols, e.g. meprobamate; and the benzodiazepines, e.g. chlordiazepoxide, diazepam, nitrazepam and several other related compounds. The chemical structures are shown in Fig. 9.1.

Although the drugs are sedative and hypnotic, which probably accounts in part for their efficacy, they probably also have a more specific anxiety-reducing action.

The barbiturates are the most dangerous of these drugs and have frequently led to abuse. The newer anxiety-reducing agents are comparatively safe.

In experimental animals, as in man, the benzodiazepines usually have a marked calming effect. However, they have been known to cause paradoxical aggression in psychotics, and occasionally the appearance of paranoic ideas. In 'normal' volunteers they have been shown to increase hostile interactions, especially when an element of frustration is introduced, and it seems likely that their effects may be altered by environmental factors. This has been clearly shown in mice where chlordiazepoxide has been shown to increase aggression and increase mortality when the animals are kept in large groups but not when housed singly or in small groups.

Muscle-relaxant actions

The muscle-relaxing properties of the minor tranquillisers may contribute to the more relaxed and tension-free feelings which they produce. These effects may be more important in uses in which they are employed as anticonvulsants. For example,

Barbiturates : see table 6.2

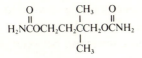

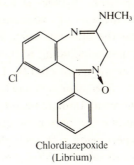

Meprobamate

Chlordiazepoxide
(Librium)

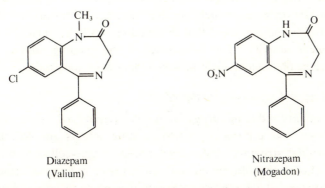

Diazepam
(Valium)

Nitrazepam
(Mogadon)

Fig. 9.1. Sedative-hypnotic and anxiety-reducing drugs.

diazepam has been considered to be the drug of choice for the
emergency treatment of status epilepticus and has also been used
successfully in the management of tetanus. However, nitrazepam
may induce major seizures or centrencephalic seizures in
epileptics.

In small doses, all of the sedative–hypnotic drugs reduce
polysynaptic spinal reflexes more than they reduce monosynaptic
reflexes. This effect may be due to a combination of pre- and
postsynaptic actions. An interesting but so far unexplained action
of barbiturates and diazepam is that they increase spinal presynaptic inhibition which may partly explain the reduction of
reflex excitability.

A component of brain homogenates has been shown to bind

strychnine, a competitive antagonist for the spinal inhibitory mediator, glycine. It has been found that the benzodiazepines in 'therapeutic' concentrations prevent strychnine binding and that the affinities correlated with a number of pharmacological actions, including a 'human bioassay', muscle relaxation and anticonvulsant effects. There was no correlation between pharmacological effects and binding to cholinergic or opiate receptors. Therefore it might be anticipated that the benzodiazepenes should modify the action of glycine or its antagonist strychnine, but experiments with iontophoretic administration have so far failed to substantiate this hypothesis. In another study of binding it has recently been shown that the benzodiazepenes bind to sites in brain homogenates which do not interact with any of the putative transmitters and that this binding is also correlated with biological activity. The relevance of the binding studies to important pharmacological actions is therefore uncertain.

Sedative and anxiety-reducing effects

The anxiety-reducing drugs alter the activity of supraspinal neurones and differences between drug effects on different supraspinal structures have been noted. Single-cell recordings have shown that diazepam and, to a lesser extent, chlordiazepoxide caused a greater reduction in the spontaneous activity of hippocampal neurones than of neurones in the pre-optic area of the hypothalamus or reticular formation and that the effect on reticular neurones was greater than that on spinal interneurones. In contrast, both meprobamate and pentobarbitone exerted their most marked effects upon neurones in the reticular formation. The hippocampus is part of the limbic system, which includes the cingulate gyrus, fornix, amygdala and hippocampus, and is considered to have an important function in behaviour and, in particular, in emotional responses. It is therefore pertinent that the benzodiazepines appear to exert their most prominent effects upon this system, as found in the studies on single neurones and in several other investigations on evoked population potentials and EEGs recorded from this area of the brain. It is also of interest that meprobamate and the barbiturates, which are also employed as anxiety-reducing drugs, appear to exert their effects at a different level of the central nervous system.

Biochemical studies have shown that the anxiety-reducing drugs produce changes in brain monoamines, especially when basic levels have been modified by stress. There is a marked increase in the turnover of noradrenaline in the brain of rats subjected to stress-inducing procedures such as immobilisation or electric shocks to the feet. This increase in turnover, revealed by changes in the incorporation of labelled noradrenaline in the brain or by measuring the level of noradrenaline after inhibition of tyrosine hydroxylase, was unaccompanied by any significant change in levels of endogenous noradrenaline. With relatively mild degrees of stress there were no detectable changes in dopamine metabolism, but the turnover of dopamine decreased when the stress was more severe.

The benzodiazepines counteracted the stress-induced increase in noradrenaline turnover. Similar effects are also produced by meprobamate and phenobarbitone and it seems likely that a decrease in impulse flow in central noradrenergic neurones may be caused by all anxiety-reducing drugs. However, this is not their only action on central catecholamine mechanisms because the benzodiazepines also decrease the resting turnover of dopamine and accentuate the fall in turnover produced by severe stress.

There is some evidence that the benzodiazepines also affect the turnover of 5-hydroxytryptamine in brain. Experiments were carried out on groups of rats injected with either a single dose of oxazepam or six doses at daily intervals. After the single or multiple injections, the animals were sacrificed and the turnover of both 5-hydroxytryptamine and noradrenaline was measured. The turnover of noradrenaline was decreased after the first dose but was not significantly different from controls after six doses. This was correlated with the sedative effect of oxazepam which was marked after a single but not after repeated injections. In contrast, the turnover of 5-hydroxytryptamine was decreased in all rats and this was correlated with a lack of tolerance to the 'anxiety-reducing' action revealed in behavioural tests in a conflict situation. These data are summarised in Table 9.1, and

Table 9.1. *Effects of oxazepam on monoamine turnover and behaviour in rats*

	After first dose	After sixth dos
NA turnover	Decreased	No effe
Sedation	Present	Absen
5-HT turnover	Decreased	Decrea:
'Anxiety-reduction'	Present	Presei

After Wise, Berger & Stein (1972).

could indicate that changes in noradrenaline metabolism n associated with sedative effects whereas a change i hydroxytryptamine metabolism may be more closely relateu more specific anxiety-reducing effects.

In conclusion, it appears that the anxiety-reducing drugs, and the benzodiazepines in particular, have a primary target for their effects in the limbic system or reticular formation, and that at the biochemical level the effect may be related to a reduction in stress-induced changes in the function of monoaminergic systems. Other actions on presynaptic inhibition and strychnine binding are more difficult to interpret but may be related to muscle-relaxant properties.

DRUGS USED IN SCHIZOPHRENIA

Range of actions

The introduction of the phenothiazine derivative chlorpromazine in the mid-1950s caused a revolution in the management of schizophrenia. Previously the only treatments available were surgical methods, convulsant or insulin-shock therapy, ECT and sedation or restraint.

Chlorpromazine is not without its drawbacks, which include sedation which is particularly evident during the early stages of treatment, extrapyramidal symptoms, a hypotensive effect, liver dysfunction, dermatological problems such as contact dermatitis and photosensitivity and more serious, but fortunately rarer, blood dyscrasias including agranulocytosis and leucopenia. In

Table 9.2. *Severity of major side-effects of antischizophrenic drugs at effective antipsychotic doses*

	Extrapyramidal symptoms	Sedative effect	Hypotensive effect
...mazine	++	+++	++(+)
...zine	+	+++	++
...mazine	+++	++	++
...perazine	+++	++	+
...idol	+++	+	+
...ine	+	+	
...de	+	0	

...empts to overcome some of these problems many similar drugs have been synthesised but chlorpromazine is still used a great deal.

In addition to the phenothiazines, antischizophrenic agents (Fig. 9.2) include: thioxanthenes, e.g. flupenthixol; butyrophenones, e.g. haloperidol and spiroperidol; diphenylbutyl piperidines, e.g. pimozide; and dibenzodiazepines, e.g. clozapine. Reserpine was also used at one time in schizophrenic patients but it may cause severe depression, sometimes leading to suicidal tendencies.

Although the drugs may differ markedly in potency, mere increases in potency are not a sufficient indication for one drug rather than another and, among the phenothiazines, it is probable that in effective doses none are more efficacious than chlorpromazine itself. The preference for one drug rather than another will therefore depend upon its spectrum of effects in various patients. Table 9.2 shows that the major side-effects of extrapyramidal symptoms, sedation and hypotension are unrelated to the antipsychotic action and we shall later attempt to explain this variation in relation to mechanism of action at the cellular level.

In addition to its antipsychotic action, chlorpromazine has a number of central effects. The sedative effect has already been noted. However, unlike the antipsychotic action which is persistent, the sedative effect becomes less marked with repeated administration and this may indicate a different mechanism. Sudden withdrawal may elicit withdrawal symptoms but there is

Phenothiazines

Chlorpromazine

Thioridazine

Butyrophenones

Haloperidol

Diphenylbutylpiperidines

Pimozide

Thioxanthenes

Flupenthixol

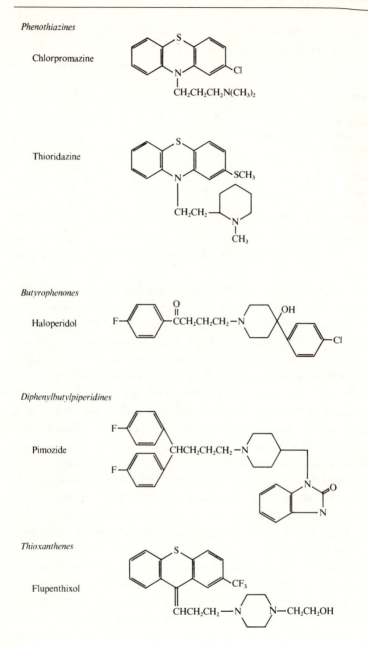

Dibenzazepines

Clozapine

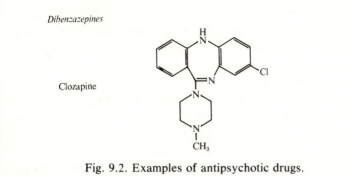

Fig. 9.2. Examples of antipsychotic drugs.

no true addiction to or craving for the drug. There is a hypothermic action, probably produced by an alteration of the set-point regulating mechanism in the hypothalamus. This effect, like many of the actions are due to a dopamine-receptor blocking action exerted in the hypothalamus. The hypothermic action has been utilised in the production of 'artificial hibernation' to reduce metabolic demands for oxygen, especially in heart surgery. Chlorpromazine is also an anti-emetic agent but its marked sedative action is a disadvantage in using it to counteract travel-sickness. The drug also potentiates the effects of other CNS depressants. This is mainly a central effect but it may also affect liver enzymes causing degradation of the drug.

Mechanisms of action

Amphetamine in high doses can cause symptoms (a toxic psychosis) reminiscent of those occurring in paranoid schizo-phrenia. In experimental animals the drug causes characteristic behavioural effects which can be counteracted by the antischizo-phrenic drugs. Amphetamine is known to cause a release of dopamine in the brain and this provided one of the first links in the chain of evidence correlating antipsychotic action with an antagonism to dopamine at the receptor level.

There are three principal dopaminergic systems of neurones in the brain (Chapter 5), the nigrostriatal, the mesolimbic and the tuberoinfundibular systems, and it is presumably the second of these which is important for the antischizophrenic effect whereas the first is linked to the occurrence of the extrapyramidal motor effects of the drugs. However, the antischizophrenic drugs also interact with noradrenergic systems.

If we consider four examples including the antipsychotic drugs chlorpromazine, haloperidol and pimozide and an antihistamine drug, promethazine, which is a phenothiazine derivative like chlorpromazine, but lacking an antipsychotic action, it has been shown that all three antischizophrenic drugs increase the turnover of dopamine in the brain, but promethazine is ineffective. However, only chlorpromazine has any marked effect on noradrenaline turnover and this is correlated with its greater sedative action. Thus it may be that the effect on noradrenergic systems is linked to the occurrence of sedative effects, whereas an effect on dopaminergic systems is essential for antipsychotic action. The effect on brain dopamine is also associated with the occurrence of extrapyramidal motor effects, but the correlation is not as good and we shall come to the explanation of this later.

Evidence for an interaction with dopamine receptors

Homovanillic acid is formed from dopamine by the combined action of monoamine oxidase and catechol-0-methyltransferase (Fig. 9.3).

Increased turnover of dopamine is therefore associated with an increased production of homovanillic acid. It has been postulated that the turnover of dopamine is regulated by a negative-feedback system in which a block of postsynaptic receptors would cause a reduction in the feedback suppression of transmitter synthesis and a consequent increase in turnover (Fig. 9.4). Chlorpromazine increases turnover. However, this is not the only mechanism regulating transmitter synthesis because it has been shown that chlorpromazine may still increase dopamine turnover after an acute lesion in the dopaminergic projection.

The antagonism by antipsychotic drugs of the behavioural actions of amphetamine is another part of the evidence that the drugs operate via effects on a dopaminergic system in the brain. More direct evidence in support of this postulate comes from biochemical studies on adenylate cyclase.

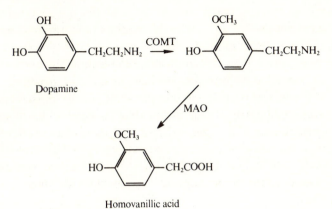

Dopamine

Homovanillic acid

Fig. 9.3. Metabolism of dopamine.

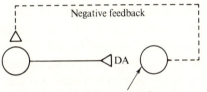

Antipsychotics block DA receptor here

Fig. 9.4. Proposed mechanism of increased DA turnover by antipsychotic drugs.

Adenylate cyclase mediates the conversion of ATP to 3′, 5′ cyclic AMP. An adenylate cyclase extracted from caudate nucleus, olfactory tubercle and nucleus accumbens of rat brain is activated by dopamine or apomorphine, considered to be a dopamine receptor agonist. The effective antipsychotic agents are particularly effective in counteracting this activating effect of dopamine on adenylate cyclase, but the rank order of their potencies for clinical and biochemical effects are similar but not identical and for a time there was no adequate explanation for this discrepancy. Thus, although α-flupenthixol is the most potent drug in both clinical and biochemical tests, the butyrophenones (e.g. haloperidol) are more potent than chlorpromazine in schizophrenia but are less potent in the biochemical test. This discrepancy may be partly due to the fact that the butyrophenones have another effect, relatively lacking in chlorpromazine, which explains their clinical effectiveness: the butyrophenones are more potent than chlorpromazine in blocking the evoked release of dopamine from nerve terminals in slices of striatum.

It has also been found that the ability of the antischizophrenic drugs to interfere with the binding of haloperidol to rat brain preparations is a better indication of their clinical effectiveness than inhibition of dopamine-stimulated adenylate cyclase. There is no adequate explanation for this fact, although it has been postulated that dopamine and its antagonists may bind at different sites.

Neurophysiological attempts to demonstrate an interaction between the dopamine receptor and antischizophrenic drugs have not been very successful. Although both chlorpromazine and α-flupenthixol administered by microelectrophoretic techniques have been shown to antagonise the action of dopamine in the putamen and amygdala, intravenous administration of the antipsychotic drugs was ineffective. Although a number of possible explanations for this failure to cause antagonism by intravenous injection could be proposed, one cannot escape the obvious paradox that in clinical use the drugs are effective when administered systemically.

One last item of evidence that the antischizophrenic drugs are well suited to an interaction with dopamine receptors comes from X-ray crystallography where it has been shown that chlorpromazine and a few other antipsychotic agents have a crystal structure, part of which corresponds very closely to the conformation of dopamine itself.

Extrapyramidal side-effects

The extrapyramidal effects of antischizophrenic drugs are most troublesome during the early stages of treatment but may sometimes be overcome more rapidly by a reduction in dose. When this is not possible due to the recurrence of schizophrenic symptoms, anti-Parkinsonian drugs, especially the cholinergic antagonists may be employed. However, L-DOPA cannot be used.

Table 9.3. *Dissociation constants of some antipsychotic drugs for binding to muscarinic and dopaminergic receptors*

	Muscarinic (M)	Dopaminergic (D)	M/D
Thioridazine	2.5×10^{-8}	1.3×10^{-7}	5.2
Clozapine	5.5×10^{-8}	1.7×10^{-7}	3.1
Pimozide	1.6×10^{-7}	1.4×10^{-7}	0.87
Chlorpromazine	3.5×10^{-7}	4.8×10^{-8}	0.14
Spiroperidol	1.2×10^{-5}	9.5×10^{-8}	0.008
Trifluoperazine	4.0×10^{-6}	1.9×10^{-8}	0.005
α-flupenthixol	2.2×10^{-6}	1.0×10^{-9}	0.0005

After Iversen (1975).

The extrapyramidal symptoms include akinesia, rigidity and tremor. Other symptoms, not seen as frequently in patients with Parkinson's disease, include akathisia, dystonia and tardive dyskinesia.

These side-effects may be attributed to a block of dopamine receptors in the neostriatum, which is innervated by the nigrostriatal dopaminergic pathway. The occurrence of extra-pyramidal effects does not correlate with the ability of the drugs to inhibit dopamine activation of adenylate cyclase; all of the antischizophrenic drugs share this action to some degree but not all produce the same severity of extrapyramidal action in equi-effective antipsychotic doses. It has recently been shown that those agents which are potent antipsychotic agents but have the lowest incidence of extrapyramidal actions, also have the greatest affinity for binding to muscarinic receptors for acetylcholine in brain. Some examples of relative affinities for dopaminergic and muscarinic receptors are shown in Table 9.3.

Those drugs at the top of the table such as thioridazine, clozapine and pimozide have a much lower incidence of extra-pyramidal effects than those at the bottom of the table.

Confirmation that these differing relative affinities for choli-nergic and dopaminergic receptors cause differential effects on the limbic and neostriatal systems has been obtained in studies of the effects of drugs on the turnover of dopamine in these two areas

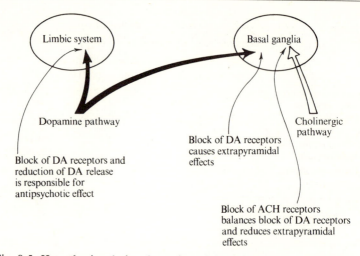

Fig. 9.5. Hypothesis relating the action of drugs in the basal ganglia and limbic system to antipsychotic action and production of motor disorders.

of the nervous system. The three antipsychotic drugs thioridazine, chlorpromazine and fluphenazine produced a similar increase in turnover of dopamine in the nucleus accumbens. However, thioridazine, which causes the least extrapyramidal symptoms and binds most strongly to muscarinic receptors, caused the least effect on dopamine turnover in the neostriatum, whereas at the other extreme, fluphenazine caused the greatest increase in turnover of dopamine in the neostriatum and caused the greatest incidence of extrapyramidal effects. This finding may be attributed to a lack of cholinergic input to the nucleus accumbens whereas in the basal ganglia, the cholinergic innervation may act as a physiological balance to the dopaminergic innervation from substantia nigra. When the control of basal ganglia activity is disturbed by a block of dopamine receptors, then motor symptoms are evident. When this disturbance is counterbalanced by a simultaneous block of the cholinergic system, then motor dysfunction is kept in abeyance. However, block of muscarinic receptors may be responsible for some of the peripheral side-effects of antipsychotic drug treatment, including dry-mouth, blurring of vision and constipation.

This hypothesis of the mechanism for the production of extrapyramidal motor disorders during drug treatment of schizophrenia is illustrated in Fig. 9.5.

DRUGS USED IN PSYCHOTIC DEPRESSION

The depressive states to be considered here include endogenous depression and manic depression. There are changes in the metabolism of catecholamines and 5-HT, in the excretion of metabolites and in the levels of metabolites in CSF in the manic and depressive phases of manic depression. This may indicate either that the basic disorder involves a malfunction of monoaminergic transmission or that such changes are the consequence rather than the cause of the disease. Regardless of whether malfunction of monoaminergic systems represents cause or effect, it is quite clear that some drugs which modify monoaminergic function have been highly successful in treating the depressive symptoms. Prior to the introduction of such drugs for the management of depressive illness, the only effective treatments were electroconvulsive therapy, pentylenetetrazole shock and insulin shock treatment. Of these older methods, only ECT persists and is still used extensively especially in those patients resistant to drug therapy.

Most currently used antidepressant drugs (Fig. 9.6) fall into two groups, those which inhibit monoamine oxidase (MAO) and those which inhibit amine uptake, e.g. imipramine. However, newer drugs which lack these properties, e.g. iprindole and mianserin, may nevertheless be antidepressant.

The mood-elevating effect of iproniazid was first noted in 1951 when it was introduced for the treatment of tuberculosis. It was subsequently shown to be an MAO inhibitor but was not tried as an antidepressant until 1957. Many such drugs have now been discovered but toxic effects on the liver, CNS and cardiovascular system have caused many of them to be withdrawn. The tricyclic antidepressants such as imipramine are less toxic and therefore more widely used. Imipramine was originally developed as a possible histamine antagonist and was then tried as a sedative in

Monoamine oxidase inhibitors

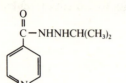

Iproniazid
(prototype)

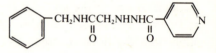

Tranylcypromine

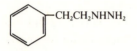

Phenelzine

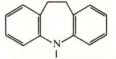

Nialamide

Tricyclic compounds

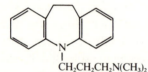

Imipramine

Desipramine

Amitriptyline

Fig. 9.6. Antidepressants.

agitated psychotic patients in 1958. However, its sedative effects are much less than those of chlorpromazine and it also differed from chlorpromazine in being particularly effective in patients with endogenous depression.

The main action of MAO inhibitors is to elevate mood in depressed patients but the effect may take some weeks to become apparent. It is tempting to attribute the therapeutic effect to

Table 9.4. *Block of amine uptake in synaptosomes by anti-depressants*

	Relative potency (imipramine = 1)	
	NA	5-HT
Desipramine	20	0.2
Amitriptyline	18	0.6
Chlorpromazine	2	0.1
Imipramine	1	1
Nortriptyline	0.8	0.2
3-Chloroimipramine	—	5.1
Iprindole	Inactive	Inactive

After Horn & Tracy (1974); Horn, A. S., Coyle, J. T. & Snyder, S. H. (1971) *Mol. Pharmacol.*, 7, 66.

inhibition of MAO which controls intraneuronal concentrations of monoamines in the cytoplasm. However, the correlation between clinical effectiveness and inhibition of MAO is not good and a further difficulty with the hypothesis is that whereas inhibition of MAO is rapid, the therapeutic effects are slow in onset. These observations do not eliminate the possibility that the drugs may act primarily via inhibition of MAO because other factors may be involved in determination of potency *in vivo* and the slow onset of clinical effects may be due to slow adaptive changes resulting from maintained inhibition of MAO, and that some of the behavioural consequences of MAO inhibition may therefore be delayed.

The tricyclic drugs may cause sedation in normal subjects but the subjective effects tend to be unpleasant. There is also a decrease in cognitive processes which may be more marked than with chlorpromazine. These effects in normal subjects may be observed after a single administration but the mood elevation in depressed patients may take weeks to develop, as with the MAO inhibitors. The subjective effects of MAO inhibitors and imipramine in depressed patients may also be somewhat different:

imipramine causes less outright euphoria but a greater attenuation of depressive thoughts than MAO inhibitors.

The most notable pharmacological action of the tricyclic antidepressants is that they block high affinity uptake mechanisms for catecholamines and 5-HT (Table 9.4). The block of re-uptake should allow more amine to be available for interaction with postsynaptic receptors, thus achieving the same result as MAO inhibition but by a different mechanism. Such an increase in postsynaptic receptor activation might be expected to result in a decreased transmitter synthesis by negative-feedback. Such a decrease in 5-HT turnover has been demonstrated after treatment with chloroimipramine, which selectively blocks 5-HT uptake.

It is not clear to what extent block of NA or block of 5-HT uptake is responsible for the antidepressant action and it will be noted in Table 9.4 that these two properties appear to be independent. This may explain the relatively poor correlation between clinical activity and block of uptake. However, there must be other ways of alleviating depression because some recently tried antidepressant drugs such as iprindole and mianserin are neither MAO inhibitors nor uptake-blockers. Nevertheless, there are indications that the primary actions may still be on aminergic systems.

Thus it appears that drugs may alleviate endogenous depression by one or a combination of actions on monoaminergic systems. It may be that the several possible types of effect may explain some of the poor correlations between clinical effectiveness and any one of these properties.

The manic phase of manic depression may be treated with phenothiazines such as chlorpromazine and antidepressants are still used to reduce the depressive symptoms. However, it has become clear that continued treatment with lithium salts may be extremely useful in the longer term management and prophylactic treatment of both manic and depressive phases.

Lithium has been in medical use, sometimes with rather dubious effects, for centuries. Its use in psychiatry began around 1950, but serious interest did not arise until about 1965. The low cost, it is one of the commonest elements in the earth's crust, did not make it an attractive commercial proposition and it did not come into general use until about 1971. In its initial use for the acute control of mania and depression it is not very effective. It is probably not very effective, if effective at all in the management of endogenous depression but comes into its own in the long-term management of manic depressives.

There is very little effect in the first 7–10 days of treatment. The plasma level cannot be allowed to rise above about 1.0 mEq/L, or, in extreme cases, 1.5 mEq/L without the production of severe side-effects. Lithium is a simple, monovalent cation, slightly larger than sodium in the hydrated state. It can diffuse across membranes in place of sodium but it is not handled efficiently by the sodium-pump. The resulting slow accumulation of lithium within cells alters membrane properties and possibly may give rise to other secondary effects.

The effects which have been attributed to lithium are diverse and not always consistent. These include stimulation of noradrenaline turnover, inhibition of 5-HT turnover, stimulation of 5-HT synthesis, inhibition of stimulus-induced amine release, stimulation or inhibition of amine uptake and changes in the levels of amine precursors and metabolites in the CSF. In addition, the uptake of choline in the erythrocytes of depressed patients on lithium treatment is markedly reduced, apparently by an unknown irreversible process. There may also be changes in cholinergic function in the CNS.

It seems reasonable at the present time to attribute all of these effects to the fact that lithium is not handled by the sodium-pump, but it does not help a great deal in understanding how any of these actions are important in the undoubted therapeutic effect in manic depression.

PSYCHOTOMIMETIC DRUGS

A variety of drugs, with a wide spectrum of pharmacological activities, can cause psychedelic effects ranging from euphoria, distortions of perceptual processes, impairment of memory, disorientation and hallucinations to delirium. Some of these sub-

Amphetamine

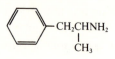

Mescaline

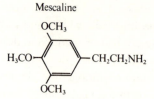

Lysergic acid diethylamide

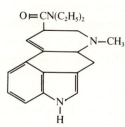

Psilocybin

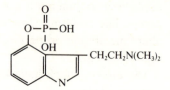

'Ditran', N-ethyl-3-piperidyl
phenylcyclopentyl glycolate

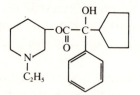

Tetrahydrocannabinol

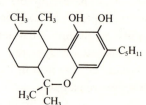

Fig. 9.7. Psychotomimetic drugs.

stances have been used for many centuries in tribal ceremonies,
e.g. mescaline from peyote, and psilocybin from mushrooms of
the *Psilocybe* species whereas others have achieved notoriety in
more recent times, e.g. lysergic acid diethylamide (LSD), amphetamine and tetrahydrocannabinol (from marihuana). Psychosis
may also be produced by drugs with atropine-like actions and may
even be seen with atropine itself in large doses. Some potent

anticholinergic drugs such as 'Ditran' (N-ethyl-3-piperidylphenyl-cyclopentylglycolate) are extremely potent psychotomimetic substances. The structures of some of these compounds are shown in Fig. 9.7.

The effects of these substances may differ markedly in different individuals and may often resemble the symptoms of schizophrenia. These differences probably reflect to a large degree the psychological make-up of the drug user, his expectations and attitudes, his social, cultural and genetic background. The variation may not be particularly greater than the bewildering array of symptoms displayed in different schizophrenic patients.

It seems probable that superficially similar behavioural effects can be produced by quite different pharmacological actions. Nevertheless, there is some common ground in that all may interfere with chemical synaptic transmission, albeit with different chemical transmitters.

Thus it is known that amphetamine releases dopamine from central dopaminergic terminals whereas the major pharmacological action of the phenylcyclopentylglycolates is an antagonism to the muscarinic action of acetylcholine.

When it was shown that LSD-25 was a powerful antagonist of 5-HT on smooth muscle in the early 1950s it seemed reasonable to speculate that this action might be the basis of its hallucinogenic effect. However, the 2-bromo derivative is also a powerful 5-HT antagonist and yet lacks the psychotomimetic effect. An alternative possibility that substances such as LSD-25 have an action like 5-HT in inhibiting the 5-HT-containing neurones of the raphé nucleus has been proposed by Aghajanian on the basis of experiments with systemic administration of small doses of LSD-25, but others have shown antagonism between LSD-25 and 5-HT at the same site by microelectrophoretic techniques. There are biochemical observations indicating that a number of psychotomimetic agents including d-LSD, mescaline, acetyl-d-LSD, psilocybin and tetrahydrocannabinol all interact with central 5-HT mechanisms. Experiments *in vitro* have shown that d-LSD, acetyl-d-LSD and mescaline inhibit the electrically evoked release of 5-HT from slices of rat brain. In other studies it has been shown

Table 9.5. *Correlation between effect and ability to inhibit 5-HT release or to raise brain levels of 5-HT*

	Psychoto-mimetic	Inhibition of noradrenaline release	Inhibition of 5-HT release or increase in brain level
d-LSD	+	+	+
1-LSD	0	0	0
Acetyl-d-LSD	+	0	+
2-Bromo-LSD	0	0	0
Psilocybin	+	?	+
Tetrahydrocannabinol	+	?	+
Mescaline	+	0	+

After Kopin, I. J. (1970) *Neurosci. Res. Prog. Bull.*, **8**, 27. Freedman, D. X. (1970) *Neurosci. Res. Prog. Bull.*, **8**, 38.
+, effective; 0, no effect; ?, effect not known.

that 5-HT levels in brain are increased by d-LSD, mescaline, psilocybin and tetrahydrocannabinol: a decreased release of 5-HT could give rise to the increased levels.

As shown in Table 9.5 although d-LSD also reduced the release of noradrenaline from brain slices, other potent psychotomimetic drugs did not. Thus, there seems to be a good correlation between ability to affect 5-HT transmission and psychotomimetic action with a number of active drugs. All of these observations may be brought together if the decreased turnover of 5-HT is due to a negative-feedback caused by a 5-HT-like depressant action of LSD-like compounds on neurones of the raphé, but this needs to be confirmed by other investigators. However, there are non-hallucinogenic LSD congeners with the same effect as LSD on neurones of the raphé.

Microelectrophoretic studies with LSD and its 2-bromo deriva-tive on cortical neurones have shown that both compounds antagonise the excitatory effect of 5-HT, whereas other inves-tigators have found that the excitatory but not the depressant actions of the 5-HT in the brainstem are antagonised by LSD but not by 2-bromo LSD. The significant action of LSD on central 5-HT neurones therefore remains to be established.

Selected reading

Chapter 1   Introduction

Goodman, L. S. & Gilman, A. (1975). *The Pharmacological Basis of Therapeutics*, 5th edn. London: Macmillan.
McLennan, H. (1970). *Synaptic transmission*, 2nd edn. Philadelphia: W. B. Saunders Co.

Chapter 2   Pharmacology of the neuromuscular junction

Colquhoun, D. (1975). Mechanisms of drug action at the voluntary muscle end plate. *Ann. Rev. Pharmacol.* 307–25.
Grob, D. (ed.) (1976). Myasthenia gravis. *Ann. N.Y. Acad. Sci.*, **274**.
Katz, B. (1966). *Nerve, Muscle and Synapse*. New York: McGraw-Hill.
Katz, B. & Miledi, R. (1972). The statistical nature of the acetylcholine potential and its molecular components. *J. Physiol.*, **224**, 665–99.
Katz, B. & Miledi, R. (1973). The characteristics of 'end-plate noise' produced by different depolarizing drugs. *J. Physiol.*, **230**, 707–17.
Lundh, H., Cull-Candy, S. G., Leander, S. & Thesleff, S. (1976). Restoration of transmitter release in botulinum-poisoned skeletal muscle. *Brain Res.*, **110**, 194–8.
Narahashi, T. (1974). Chemicals as tools in the study of excitable membranes. *Physiol. Rev.*, **54**, 813–89.
Neher, E. & Sakman, B. (1976). Single channel currents recorded from membrane of denervated frog muscle fibres. *Nature*, **260**, 799–802.
Rang, H. P. (1973). Receptor mechanisms. *Br. J. Pharmacol.*, **48**, 475–95.
Rang, H. P. & Ritter, J. M. (1970). On the mechanism of desensitization at cholinergic receptors. *Mol.: Pharmacol.*, **6**, 357–83.
Rang, H. P. & Ritter, J. M. (1970). The relationship between desensitization and the metaphilic effect at cholinergic receptors. *Mol. Pharmacol.*, **6**, 383–90.
Thesleff, S. (1955). The mode of neuromuscular block caused by acetylcholine, nicotine, decamethonium and succinylcholine. *Acta Physiol. Scand.*, **34**, 218–31.

Chapter 3   Pharmacology of the autonomic nervous system

Dollery, C. T. (1973). Adrenergic drugs in the treatment of hypertension. *Br. Med. Bull.*, **29**, 158–62.
Eccles, R. M. & Libet, B. (1961). Origin and blockade of the synaptic responses of curarized sympathetic ganglia. *J. Physiol.*, **157**, 484–503.

Goodman, L. S. & Gilman, A. (1975). *The Pharmacological Basis of Therapeutics*, 5th edn. London: Macmillan.

Kebabian, J. W. & Greengard, P. (1971). Dopamine-sensitive adenyl cyclase: Possible role in synaptic transmission. *Science*, **174**, 1346–8.

Langer, S. Z. (1977). Presynaptic receptors and their role in the regulation of transmitter release. *Br. J. Pharmacol.*, **60**, 481–97.

Laverty, R. (1973). The mechanisms of action of some anti-hypertensive drugs. *Br. Med. Bull.*, **29**, 152–7.

Libet, B. (1977). The role SIF cells play in ganglionic transmission. *Adv. in Biochem. Psychopharmacol.*, **16**, 541–6.

Volle, R. (1969). Ganglionic transmission. *Ann. Rev. Pharmacol.*, **9**, 135–47.

Chapter 4   Techniques used to study transmitters and drug action in the CNS

Iversen, S. D. & Iversen, L. L. (1975). *Behavioural Pharmacology*. Oxford University Press.

Kelly, J. S. (1975). Microiontophoretic application of drugs onto single neurones. In *Handbook of Psychopharmacology*, eds. Iversen, L. L., Iversen, S. D. & Snyder, S. H., vol. 2, pp. 29–67. New York & London: Plenum Press.

Nastuk, W. L. (ed.) (1964). *Physical Techniques in Biological Research*, vol. 6. *Electrophysiological Methods*. New York & London: Academic Press.

Chapter 5   Central neurotransmitters

Cooper, J. R., Bloom, F. E. & Roth, R. H. (1974). *The Biochemical Basis of Neuropharmacology*. Oxford University Press.

Curtis, D. R. & Johnston, G. A. R. (1974). Amino acid transmitters in the mammalian central nervous system. *Ergebn. Physiol.* **69**, 98–188.

Curtis, D. R. & Ryall, R. W. (1966). The synaptic excitation of Renshaw cells. *Exptl Brain Res.*, **2**, 81–96.

Green, A. R. & Grahame-Smith, D. G. (1975). 5-Hydroxytryptamine and other indoles in the central nervous system. In *Handbook of Psychopharmacology*, ed. Iversen, L. L., Iversen, S. D. & Snyder, S.H., vol. 3, pp. 169–245. New York & London: Plenum Press.

Kelly, J. S. & Beart, P. M. (1975). Amino acid receptors in CNS. II GABA in supraspinal regions. In *Handbook of Psychopharmacology*, ed. Iversen, L. L., Iversen, S. D. & Snyder, S. H., vol. 4. New York & London: Plenum Press.

Krnjevic, K. (1974). Chemical nature of synaptic transmission in vertebrates. *Physiol. Rev.*, **54**, 418–540.

Livett, B. G. (1973). Histochemical visualization of peripheral and central adrenergic neurones. *Br. Med. Bull.*, **29**, 93–9.

Phillis, J. W. (1970). *The Pharmacology of Synapses*. Oxford: Pergamon Press.

Ryall, R. W. (1970). Renshaw cell mediated inhibition of Renshaw cells: Patterns of excitation and inhibition from impulses in motor axon collaterals. *J. Neurophysiol.* **33**, 257–70.

Ryall, R. W. (1975). Amino acid receptors in the CNS. I GABA and glycine in spinal cord. In *Handbook of Psychopharmacology*, ed. Iversen, L. L., Iversen, S. D. & Snyder, S. H., vol., 4, pp. 83–128. New York & London: Plenum Press.

Snyder, S. H. (1975). The glycine receptor in the mammalian central nervous system. *Br. J. Pharmacol.*, **53**, 473–84.

Von Euler, U. S. & Pernow, B. (eds.) (1976). *Substance P.* New York: Raven Press.

Chapter 6   General anaesthetics

Dundee, J. W. (1971). Comparative analysis of intravenous anaesthetics. *Anesthesiology*, **35**, 137–48.

Dundee, J. W. & Haslett, W. H. K. (1970). The benzodiazepines: A review of their actions and uses relative to anaesthetic practice. *Br. J. Anaesth.*, **42**, 217–34.

Pender, J. W. (1971). Dissociative anesthesia. *J. Am. Med. Ass.*, **215**, 1126–30.

Richards, C. D. & Hesketh, T. R. (1975). Implications for theories of anaesthesia of antagonism between anaesthetic and non-anaesthetic steroids. *Nature*, **256**, 179–82.

Seeman, P. (1972). The membrane actions of anesthetics and tranquilizers. *Pharmacol. Rev.*, **24**, 583–655.

Smith, E. B. (1974). In *Molecular Mechanisms in General Anaesthesia*, ed. Halsey *et al.* Edinburgh: Churchill-Livingstone.

Weakly, J. N. (1969). Effect of barbiturates on 'Quantal' synaptic transmission in spinal motoneurones. *J. Physiol.*, **204**, 63–77.

Chapter 7   Pharmacological control of pain

Hoffman, P. L., Walter, R. & Bulat, M. (1977). An enzymatically stable peptide with activity in the central nervous system: its penetration through the blood–CSF barrier. *Brain Res.*, **122**, 87–94.

Jessell, T. M. & Iversen, L. L. (1977). Opiate analgesics inhibit substance P release from rat trigeminal nucleus. *Nature*, **268**, 549–51.

Kosterlitz, H. W. (ed.) (1976). *Opiates and Endogenous Opioid Peptides.* Amsterdam: North-Holland Publishing Co.

Lord, J. A. H., Waterfield, A. A., Hughes, J. & Kosterlitz, H. W. (1977). Endogenous opioid peptides: multiple agonists and receptors. *Nature*, **267**, 495–9.

Mayer, D. J., Price, D. D. & Rafii, A. (1977). Antagonism of acupuncture analgesia in man by the narcotic antagonist naloxone. *Brain Res.*, **121**, 368–72.

Melzack, R. (1973). *The Puzzle of Pain.* Harmondsworth: Penguin.

Milton, A. S. (1976). Modern views on the pathogenesis of fever and the mode of action of antipyretic drugs. *J. Pharm. Pharmacol.*, **28**, 393–9.

Nathan, P. W. (1976). The gate-control theory of pain – A critical review. *Brain*, **99**, 123–58.

Pomeranz, B. (1977). Brain opiates at work in acupuncture. *New Scientist*, 6th June, 12–13.

Potter, D. R. & Payne, J. P. (1970). Newer analgesics with special reference to pentazocine. *Br. J. Anaesth.*, **42**, 186–93.

Roemar, D., Buescher, H. H., Hill, R. C., Pless, J., Bauer,. W., Cardinaux, F., Closse, A., Hauser, D. & Huguenin, R. (1977). A synthetic enkephalin analogue with prolonged parenteral and oral analgesic activity. *Nature*, **268**, 547–9.

Snyder, S. H. (1975). The opiate receptor. *Neurosci. Res. Progr. Bull.*, **13**, suppl. 1–27.

Chapter 8 Drugs and disorders of movement

Bird, E. D. & Iversen, L. L. (1974). Huntington's chorea. Post-mortem measurement of glutamic acid decarboxylase, choline acetyltransferase and dopamine in basal ganglia. *Brain*, **97**, 457–72.

Carter, C. H. & Gustafson, S. R. (1965). *Drugs in Neurospastic Disorders*. Springfield, Illinois: C. C. Thomas.

Hornykiewicz, O. (1973). Dopamine in the basal ganglia: its role and therapeutic implications (including the clinical use of L-DOPA). *Br. Med. Bull.*, **29**, 172–8.

Hornykiewicz, O. (1973). Parkinson's disease from brain homogenate to treatment. *Fed. Proc.*, **32**, 183–90.

Kanazawa, I., Bird, E., O'Connell, R. & Powell, D. (1977). Evidence for a decrease of substance P content of substantia nigra in Huntington's chorea. *Brain Res.*, **120**, 387–92.

Marks, J. (1974). The treatment of Parkinsonism with L-DOPA. Lancaster: MTP (Medical & Technical Publishing Co., Ltd).

Miller, R., Horn, A., Iversen, L. & Pinder, R. (1974). Effects of dopamine-like drugs on rat striatal adenyl cyclase have implications for CNS dopamine receptor topography. *Nature*, **250**, 238–41.

Von Voigtlander, P. F. & Moore, K. E. (1971). Dopamine: Release from the brain in vivo by amantadine. *Science*, **174**, 408–10.

Von Voigtlander, P. F. & Moore, K. E. (1973). Turning behaviour of mice with unilateral 6-hydroxydopamine lesions in the striatum: Effects of apomorphine, L-DOPA, amantadine, amphetamine and other psychomotor stimulants. *Neuropharmacol.*, **12**, 451–62.

Chapter 9 Drugs and mental disorders

Andén, N. E. & Stock, G. (1973). Effect of clozapine on the turnover of dopamine in the corpus striatum and in the limbic system. *J. Pharm. Pharmac.*, **25**, 346–8.

Berger, F. M. (1972). Social implications of psychotropic drugs. *Adv. Pharmacol. Chemother.*, **10**, 105–18.

Crow, T. J., Johnstone, E. C., Deakin, J. F. W. & Longden, A. (1976). Dopamine and schizophrenia. *The Lancet*, 11 Sept., 563–6.

Gershon, S. & Shopsin, B. (1973). *Lithium: Its Role in Psychiatric Research and Treatment.* New York & London: Plenum Press.

Horn, A. S. (1975). Structure – activity relations for neurotransmitter receptor agonists and antagonists. In *Handbook of Psychopharmacology*, ed. Iversen, L. L., Iversen, S. D. & Snyder, S. H., vol. 2, pp. 179–243. New York & London: Plenum Press.

Horn, A. S. & Tracy, R. C. A. M. (1974). Structure – activity relations for the inhibition of 5-hydroxytryptamine uptake by tricyclic antidepressants into synaptosomes from serotoninergic neurones in rat brain homogenates. *Brit. J. Pharmac.*, **51**, 399–404.

Iversen, L. L. (1975). How do antipsychotics work? *Neurosci. Res. Progr. Bull.*, **13**, suppl. 29–51.

Lader, M. H. (1976). How tranquillizers work. *Br. J. Hosp. Med.*, Dec., 622–8.

Miller, R. & Hiley, R. (1974). Antimuscarinic properties of neuroleptics and drug-induced Parkinsonism. *Nature*, **248**, 596–7.

Miller, R. J., Horn, A. S. & Iversen, L. L. (1974). The action of neuroleptic drugs on dopamine-stimulated adenosine-cyclic 3′,5′-monophosphate production in rat neostriatum and limbic forebrain. *Mol. Pharmacol.*, **10**, 759–66.

Schallek, W., Schlosser, W. & Randall, C. O. (1974). Recent developments in the pharmacology of the benzodiazepines. *Adv. Pharmacol. Chemother.*, **10**, 120–83.

Schildkraut, J. J. (1973). Neuropharmacology of the affective disorders. *Ann. Rev. Pharmacol.*, **13**, 427–54.

Smythies, J. R. (ed.) (1970). The mode of action of psychotomimetic drugs. *Neurosci. Res. Progr. Bull.* **8**, 1–149.

Squires, R. F. & Braestrup, C. (1977). Benzodiazepine receptors in rat brain. *Nature*, **266**, 732–4.

Taylor, K. M. & Laverty, R. (1969). The effect of chlordiazepoxide, diazepam and nitrazepam on catecholamine metabolism in regions of the brain. *Europ. J. Pharmacol.*, **8**, 296.

Wells, B. (1973). *Psychedelic Drugs.* Harmondsworth: Penguin.

Wise, C. D., Berger, B. D. & Stein, L. (1972). Benzodiazepines: Anxiety-reducing activity by reduction of serotonin turnover in the brain. *Science*, **177**, 180–3.

Young, A. B., Zukin, D. R. & Snyder, S. H. (1974). Interaction of benzodiazepines with central nervous glycine receptors: Possible mechanism of action. *Proc. Nat. Acad. Sci.*, **71**, 2246–50.

Index

Page numbers in italic refer to figures.

139